THE EMOTION REGULATION SKILLS SYSTEM WORKBOOK

The Emotion Regulation Skills System Workbook

A DBT-Informed Approach

SECOND EDITION

Julie F. Brown

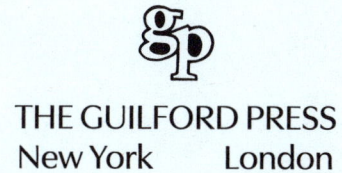

THE GUILFORD PRESS
New York   London

Copyright © 2026 Julie F. Brown
Published by The Guilford Press
A Division of Guilford Publications, Inc.
www.guilford.com

All rights reserved

Except as indicated, no part of this book may be reproduced, translated, stored in a retrieval system, or transmitted, in any form or by any means, electronic, mechanical, photocopying, microfilming, recording, or otherwise, without written permission from the publisher.

Printed in the United States of America

For product and safety concerns within the EU, please contact *GPSR@taylorandfrancis.com*,
Taylor & Francis Verlag GmbH, Kaufingerstraße 24, 80331 München, Germany.

Last digit is print number: 9 8 7 6 5 4 3 2 1

LIMITED DUPLICATION LICENSE

These materials are intended for use only under the supervision of qualified mental health professionals.

The publisher grants to individual purchasers of this book nonassignable permission to reproduce all materials for which photocopying permission is specifically granted in a footnote. This license is limited to you, the individual purchaser, for personal use or use with clients. This license does not grant the right to reproduce these materials for resale, redistribution, electronic display, or any other purposes (including but not limited to books, pamphlets, articles, video or audio recordings, blogs, file-sharing sites, internet or intranet sites, and handouts or slides for lectures, workshops, or webinars, whether or not a fee is charged). Permission to reproduce these materials for these and any other purposes must be obtained in writing from the Permissions Department of Guilford Publications.

This publication is intended to provide helpful and informative material. It is not intended to diagnose, treat, cure, or prevent any health problem or condition, nor is it intended to replace the advice of a health professional. No action should be taken based solely on the contents of this book. Always consult your physician or qualified health care professional on any matters regarding your health and before adopting any suggestions in this book or drawing inferences from it.

The author and publisher specifically disclaim all responsibility for any liability, loss, or risk, personal or otherwise, which is incurred as a consequence, directly or indirectly, from the use or application of any contents of this book.

Any and all product names referenced within this book are the trademarks of their respective owners. Always read all information provided by the manufacturers' product labels before using their products. The author and publisher are not responsible for claims made by manufacturers.

ISBN 978-1-4625-5951-0 (paperback) — ISBN 978-1-4625-5952-7 (hardcover)

About the Author

Julie F. Brown, MSW, PhD, is the president of Skills System, LLC. She is an independent social worker who has practiced in the intellectual disabilities field since the 1990s. Dr. Brown has been a dialectical behavior therapy (DBT) trainer with Behavioral Tech Institute since 2005.

Acknowledgments

As I reflect on my journey with the Skills System and how this second edition has evolved, I recall what seems like hundreds of small and large contributions people have made. At the top of the list are the individuals whom I had in skills groups, who partnered with me to create the Skills System skills. We all grappled with the concepts of dialectical behavior therapy (DBT), working to increase accessibility, reduce cognitive load, and facilitate generalization of skills. Developing the Skills System was a Partnership New-Me Activity!

My journey with The Guilford Press has been pivotal. After three painful rejections over several years, I finally was able to get the Skills System material in a form such that Kitty Moore, Publisher, was able to see the Skills System's potential. Her willingness to remain engaged though this 15-year-plus process has led to three books. I am also grateful to Katherine Sommer, who edited this book and the accompanying second-edition manual, *The Emotion Regulation Skills System for Clients with Cognitive Challenges,* for her amazing focus and dedication to improving these resources.

The work of Marsha M. Linehan, PhD, the developer of DBT, provided important foundational information for the Skills System. I would like to extend a special acknowledgment to Cynthia Sanderson, PhD, for her mentoring and support. James J. Gross, PhD, offered valuable feedback that improved the model.

Finally, I would like to acknowledge the contribution of my family to this project. My husband, children, and grandchildren have informed my work in many important ways.

I am grateful to you all.

Contents

Introduction: How to Use This Book — 1

Pre-Learning — 3

Pre-Learning, Worked Example 1: Getting to Know Me — 5
Pre-Learning, Worksheet 1: Getting to Know Me — 6
Pre-Learning, Worked Example 2: Getting to Know My Feelings — 7
Pre-Learning, Worksheet 2: Getting to Know My Feelings — 8
Pre-Learning, Worked Example 3: My New-Me and My Old-Me — 9
Pre-Learning, Worksheet 3: My New-Me and My Old-Me — 10
Pre-Learning, Worked Example 4: My Goals — 11
Pre-Learning, Worksheet 4: My Goals — 12
Pre-Learning, Worked Example 5: Exploring My Goals — 13
Pre-Learning, Worksheet 5: Exploring My Goals — 14
Pre-Learning, Worked Example 6: Exploring Targets to Reach My Goal — 15
Pre-Learning, Worksheet 6: Exploring Targets to Reach My Goal — 16

Are You Ready to Learn Skills? — 17

Learning Skills — 19

Skills List

Learning Skills, Skills List, Handout 1: Nine Core Skills — 23
Learning Skills, Skills List, Handout 2: How Our Skills Help Us — 24
Learning Skills, Skills List, Worksheet 1: Name the Skill by Picture — 25

Learning Skills, Skills List, Worksheet 2: Match the Skill Number and Initials to the Picture — 26

Learning Skills, Skills List, Worksheet 3: Name the Skill by Number — 27

System Tools

Learning Skills, System Tools, Handout 1: How I Use the Skills System — 31

Learning Skills, System Tools, Handout 2: Feelings Rating Scale with Pictures — 32

Learning Skills, System Tools, Handout 3: Feelings Rating Scale with Descriptions — 33

Learning Skills, System Tools, Worked Example 1: Feelings Rating Scale — 34

Learning Skills, System Tools, Worksheet 1: Feelings Rating Scale — 35

Learning Skills, System Tools, Handout 4: Categories of Skills — 36

Learning Skills, System Tools, Worksheet 2: Name the Skills and Categories of Skills — 37

Learning Skills, System Tools, Worked Example 2: Select the Category of Skills by Feelings Level — 38

Learning Skills, System Tools, Worksheet 3: Select the Category of Skills by Feelings Level — 39

Learning Skills, System Tools, Worksheet 4: Feelings Ratings and Categories of Skills — 40

Learning Skills, System Tools, Handout 5: Recipe for Skills — 41

Learning Skills, System Tools, Worked Example 3: Recipe for Skills—Choose How Many Skills to Use — 42

Learning Skills, System Tools, Worksheet 5: Recipe for Skills—Choose How Many Skills to Use — 43

Learning Skills, System Tools, Worksheet 6: Build Your Recipe for Skills — 44

Learning Skills, System Tools, Worked Example 4: Week 2 Practice Activity — 45

Learning Skills, System Tools, Worksheet 7: Week 2 Practice Activity — 46

Learning Skills, System Tools: Review Questions — 47

Clear Picture

Learning Skills, Clear Picture: Summary Sheet — 51

Learning Skills, Clear Picture, Handout 1: Clear Picture Do's — 52

Learning Skills, Clear Picture, Worked Example 1: Getting a Clear Picture — 53

Learning Skills, Clear Picture, Worksheet 1: Getting a Clear Picture — 54

Learning Skills, Clear Picture, Worksheet 2: Notice My Breath — 55

Learning Skills, Clear Picture, Handout 2: Notice Surroundings — 56

Learning Skills, Clear Picture, Worked Example 2: Notice Surroundings — 57

Learning Skills, Clear Picture, Worksheet 3: Notice Surroundings — 58

Learning Skills, Clear Picture, Worked Example 3: Body Check — 59

Learning Skills, Clear Picture, Worksheet 4: Body Check — 60

Learning Skills, Clear Picture, Worked Example 4: Body Check—Sensations by Feelings Level	61
Learning Skills, Clear Picture, Worksheet 5: Body Check—Sensations by Feelings Level	62
Learning Skills, Clear Picture, Handout 3: Label and Rate Feelings—List of Feelings and Emotions	63
Learning Skills, Clear Picture, Handout 4: Label and Rate Feelings—How Feelings Affect Me	64
Learning Skills, Clear Picture, Worked Example 5: Label and Rate Feelings in Specific Situations	65
Learning Skills, Clear Picture, Worksheet 6: Label and Rate Feelings in Specific Situations	66
Learning Skills, Clear Picture, Handout 5: Noticing My Thoughts	67
Learning Skills, Clear Picture, Worked Example 6: Situations That Lead to Noticing Thoughts	68
Learning Skills, Clear Picture, Worksheet 7: Situations That Lead to Noticing Thoughts	69
Learning Skills, Clear Picture, Worked Example 7: Noticing Thoughts at Different Feelings Levels	70
Learning Skills, Clear Picture, Worksheet 8: Noticing Thoughts at Different Feelings Levels	71
Learning Skills, Clear Picture, Worked Example 8: Thoughts and Feelings Lead to Urges	72
Learning Skills, Clear Picture, Worksheet 9: Thoughts and Feelings Lead to Urges	73
Learning Skills, Clear Picture, Worked Example 9: Feelings and Their Action Urges	74
Learning Skills, Clear Picture, Worksheet 10: Feelings and Their Action Urges	75
Learning Skills, Clear Picture, Worked Example 10: Action Urges by Feelings Level	76
Learning Skills, Clear Picture, Worksheet 11: Action Urges by Feelings Level	77
Learning Skills, Clear Picture, Worked Example 11: Situations That Lead to Noticing Urges	78
Learning Skills, Clear Picture, Worksheet 12: Situations That Lead to Noticing Urges	79
Learning Skills, Clear Picture, Worked Example 12: Noticing My Reactions	80
Learning Skills, Clear Picture, Worksheet 13: Noticing My Reactions	81

On-Track Thinking

Learning Skills, On-Track Thinking: Summary Sheet	85
Learning Skills, On-Track Thinking, Handout 1: On-Track Thinking to Meet My Goals	86
Learning Skills, On-Track Thinking, Worked Example 1: On-Track Thinking Through a Situation	87
Learning Skills, On-Track Thinking, Worksheet 1: On-Track Thinking Through a Situation	88

Learning Skills, On-Track Thinking, Worksheet 2: Check It — 89
Learning Skills, On-Track Thinking, Worked Example 2: Turn It — 90
Learning Skills, On-Track Thinking, Worksheet 3: Turn It — 91
Learning Skills, On-Track Thinking, Worked Example 3: On-Track Thinking—Create a Skills Plan — 92
Learning Skills, On-Track Thinking, Worksheet 4: On-Track Thinking—Create a Skills Plan — 93
Learning Skills, On-Track Thinking, Worked Example 4: Cheerleading—Blast It — 94
Learning Skills, On-Track Thinking, Worksheet 5: Cheerleading—Blast It — 95
Learning Skills, On-Track Thinking, Worked Example 5: Using Skills in My Life — 96
Learning Skills, On-Track Thinking, Worksheet 6: Using Skills in My Life — 97
Learning Skills, On-Track Thinking, Worked Example 6: Pros and Cons of Using Skills — 98
Learning Skills, On-Track Thinking, Worksheet 7: Pros and Cons of Using Skills — 99

On-Track Action

Learning Skills, On-Track Action: Summary Sheet — 103
Learning Skills, On-Track Action, Handout 1: On- and Off-Tracks — 104
Learning Skills, On-Track Action, Handout 2: Five Types of On-Track Actions — 105
Learning Skills, On-Track Action, Handout 3: Take a Step toward My Goal in Wise Mind — 106
Learning Skills, On-Track Action, Worked Example 1: On-Track Actions and My Goals — 107
Learning Skills, On-Track Action, Worksheet 1: On-Track Actions and My Goals — 108
Learning Skills, On-Track Action, Handout 4: Switch Tracks to On-Track Action — 109
Learning Skills, On-Track Action, Worked Example 2: On-Track Action—Switching Tracks — 110
Learning Skills, On-Track Action, Worksheet 2: On-Track Action—Switching Tracks — 111
Learning Skills, On-Track Action, Handout 5: On-Track Action Plans — 112
Learning Skills, On-Track Action, Worked Example 3: My On-Track Action Plan — 113
Learning Skills, On-Track Action, Worksheet 3: My On-Track Action Plan — 114
Learning Skills, On-Track Action, Worksheet 4: Balancing in My Life — 115
Learning Skills, On-Track Action, Worked Example 4: Balancing My Life — 116
Learning Skills, On-Track Action, Worksheet 5: Balancing My Life — 117
Learning Skills, On-Track Action, Handout 6: Accepting the Situation — 118
Learning Skills, On-Track Action, Handout 7: Turn the Page — 119
Learning Skills, On-Track Action, Worked Example 5: Accept the Situation and Turn the Page — 120
Learning Skills, On-Track Action, Worksheet 6: Accept the Situation and Turn the Page — 121

Learning Skills, On-Track Action, Worked Example 6: Examples of On-Track Actions	122
Learning Skills, On-Track Action, Worksheet 7: Examples of On-Track Actions	123
Learning Skills, On-Track Action, Worksheet 8: 123 Wise Mind	124

Safety Plan

Learning Skills, Safety Plan: Summary Sheet	127
Learning Skills, Safety Plan, Handout 1: Inside and Outside Risks	128
Learning Skills, Safety Plan, Worked Example 1: Examples of Inside and Outside Risks	129
Learning Skills, Safety Plan, Worksheet 1: Examples of Inside and Outside Risks	130
Learning Skills, Safety Plan, Handout 2: Getting a Clear Picture of the Risk—Three Levels of Risk	131
Learning Skills, Safety Plan, Worked Example 2: Examples of High, Medium, and Low Risks	132
Learning Skills, Safety Plan, Worksheet 2: Examples of High, Medium, and Low Risks	133
Learning Skills, Safety Plan, Handout 3: Three Types of Safety Plans	134
Learning Skills, Safety Plan, Handout 4: Three Ways to Handle Risk	135
Learning Skills, Safety Plan, Worksheet 3: Building a Safety Plan	136
Learning Skills, Safety Plan, Worked Example 3: Written Safety Plan	137
Learning Skills, Safety Plan, Worksheet 4: Written Safety Plan	138
Learning Skills, Safety Plan, Worked Example 4: Detailed Safety Plan	139
Learning Skills, Safety Plan, Worksheet 5: Detailed Safety Plan	140

New-Me Activities

Learning Skills, New-Me Activities: Summary Sheet	143
Learning Skills, New-Me Activities, Handout 1: Types of New-Me Activities	144
Learning Skills, New-Me Activities, Handout 2: Solo and Partnership New-Me Activities	145
Learning Skills, New-Me Activities, Handout 3: Focus New-Me Activities	146
Learning Skills, New-Me Activities, Worksheet 1: My Focus New-Me Activities	147
Learning Skills, New-Me Activities, Exercise 1: Body Check as a Focus New-Me Activity	148
Learning Skills, New-Me Activities, Handout 4: Feel Good New-Me Activities	149
Learning Skills, New-Me Activities, Worksheet 2: My Feel Good New-Me Activities	150
Learning Skills, New-Me Activities, Handout 5: Distraction New-Me Activities	151
Learning Skills, New-Me Activities, Worksheet 3: My Distraction New-Me Activities	152
Learning Skills, New-Me Activities, Handout 6: Fun New-Me Activities	153

Learning Skills, New-Me Activities, Worksheet 4: My Fun New-Me Activities   154

Learning Skills, New-Me Activities, Worked Example 1: Solo New-Me Activities and Self-Care   155

Learning Skills, New-Me Activities, Worksheet 5: Solo New-Me Activities and Self-Care   156

Problem Solving

Learning Skills, Problem Solving: Summary Sheet   159

Learning Skills, Problem Solving, Worked Example 1: Quick Fix   160

Learning Skills, Problem Solving, Worksheet 1: Quick Fix   161

Learning Skills, Problem Solving, Handout 1: Problem Solving   162

Learning Skills, Problem Solving, Worked Example 2A: Clear Picture of the Problem   163

Learning Skills, Problem Solving, Worksheet 2A: Clear Picture of the Problem   164

Learning Skills, Problem Solving, Worked Example 2B: Check All Options   165

Learning Skills, Problem Solving, Worksheet 2B: Check All Options   166

Learning Skills, Problem Solving, Worked Example 2C: Make Plans A, B, and C   167

Learning Skills, Problem Solving, Worksheet 2C: Make Plans A, B, and C   168

Learning Skills, Problem Solving, Worked Example 3: Problem Solving Plan   169

Learning Skills, Problem Solving, Worksheet 3: Problem Solving Plan   170

Expressing Myself

Learning Skills, Expressing Myself: Summary Sheet   173

Learning Skills, Expressing Myself, Handout 1: What Is Expressing Myself?   174

Learning Skills, Expressing Myself, Worked Example 1: Expressing What's On My Mind and In My Heart   175

Learning Skills, Expressing Myself, Worksheet 1: Expressing What's On My Mind and In My Heart   176

Learning Skills, Expressing Myself, Handout 2: Why Do I Express Myself?   177

Learning Skills, Expressing Myself, Handout 3: How Do I Use Expressing Myself?   178

Learning Skills, Expressing Myself, Handout 4: When Do I Use Expressing Myself?   179

Learning Skills, Expressing Myself, Worksheet 2: Expressing Myself Self-Check   180

Learning Skills, Expressing Myself, Worked Example 2: Expressing Myself Plan   181

Learning Skills, Expressing Myself, Worksheet 3: Expressing Myself Plan   182

Getting It Right

Learning Skills, Getting It Right: Summary Sheet   185

Learning Skills, Getting It Right, Handout 1: Getting What I Want!   186

Learning Skills, Getting It Right, Handout 2: Right Mind	187
Learning Skills, Getting It Right, Worksheet 1: Right Mind Self-Check	188
Learning Skills, Getting It Right, Handout 3: Right Person	189
Learning Skills, Getting It Right, Handout 4: Right Time and Place	190
Learning Skills, Getting It Right, Handout 5: Right Tone	191
Learning Skills, Getting It Right, Handout 6: Right Words—SEALS	192
Learning Skills, Getting It Right, Worked Example 1: Getting It Right Plan	193
Learning Skills, Getting It Right, Worksheet 2: Getting It Right Plan	194

Relationship Care

Learning Skills, Relationship Care: Summary Sheet	197
Learning Skills, Relationship Care, Handout 1: Building, Balancing, and Changing Relationships	199
Learning Skills, Relationship Care, Handout 2: Building On-Track Relationships	200
Learning Skills, Relationship Care, Worksheet 1: Building On-Track Relationships	201
Learning Skills, Relationship Care, Handout 3: Building On-Track Relationships— Different Types of Relationships	202
Learning Skills, Relationship Care, Handout 4: Balancing On-Track Relationships	203
Learning Skills, Relationship Care, Handout 5: Balancing On-Track Relationships— One- and Two-Way Streets	204
Learning Skills, Relationship Care, Worksheet 2: Balancing On-Track Relationships	205
Learning Skills, Relationship Care, Handout 6: Changing Off-Track Relationships	206
Learning Skills, Relationship Care, Worked Example 1: Relationship Check	207
Learning Skills, Relationship Care, Worksheet 3: Relationship Check	208
Learning Skills, Relationship Care, Handout 7: Finding Middle Ground	209
Learning Skills, Relationship Care, Worked Example 2: Finding Middle Ground Plan	210
Learning Skills, Relationship Care, Worksheet 4: Finding Middle Ground Plan	211
Learning Skills, Relationship Care, Handout 8: Changing Off-Track Relationships	212
Learning Skills, Relationship Care, Worked Example 3: Steps of Responsibility	213
Learning Skills, Relationship Care, Worksheet 5: Steps of Responsibility	214

Using Skills in My Life

Learning Skills, Using Skills in My Life: Skills Quiz	217
Learning Skills, Using Skills in My Life: Skills Quiz Answer Sheet	218
Learning Skills, Using Skills in My Life: Skills Plan Map	219
Learning Skills, Using Skills in My Life, Worksheet 1: Using My Skills	220
Learning Skills, Using Skills in My Life, Worksheet 2: Using My Skills	223
Learning Skills, Using Skills in My Life: Skills Certificate	225

Reaching Goals — 227

Reaching Goals, Worked Example 1: My Skills Plan — *229*
Reaching Goals, Worksheet 1: My Skills Plan — *230*
Reaching Goals, Worked Example 2: My Diary Card — *231*
Reaching Goals, Worksheet 2: My Diary Card — *232*
Reaching Goals, Worked Example 3: My Progress — *233*
Reaching Goals, Worksheet 3: My Progress — *234*
Reaching Goals, Worked Example 4: Back-Track — *235*
Reaching Goals, Worksheet 4: Back-Track — *236*
Reaching Goals, Worked Example 5: Re-Track — *237*
Reaching Goals, Worksheet 5: Re-Track — *238*

Index — 239

THE EMOTION REGULATION SKILLS SYSTEM WORKBOOK

Introduction

How to Use This Book

Hello! This is Julie, the author of the Skills System. I would like to welcome you to *The Emotion Regulation Skills System Workbook!*

The handouts and worksheets in this book are designed to help you learn how to manage feelings and reach your goals. People of all ages and abilities learn the Skills System. We all need skills to handle life's ups and downs—*I know I do!*

The Skills System is designed to be easy to learn, which helps us remember our skills when we need them. When we learn and practice skills while we are calm and thinking clearly, we will know how to use them when we are not calm and really need them. When we REALLY know skills, we can use them even when we are experiencing strong feelings.

Some people complete the *Skills System Workbook* with help from a skills instructor, therapist, family member, or other kind of support provider; others complete it independently. Some people start at the beginning and do all of the activities, while others may pick and choose specific handouts and worksheets to do. The materials in the *Skills System Workbook* are presented in the order that they are likely to be done in Skills System instruction. You can create your own learning journey and go at your own pace.

You will notice that there are three types of activities in this workbook:

- *Handouts:* Handouts explain skills concepts.

- *Worked examples:* Worked examples are completed versions of the worksheets. These have made-up information that helps us understand the concepts. The worked examples give you an example of how to fill in the worksheet. It is helpful to read the worked examples before completing the worksheets.

- *Worksheets:* Worksheets ask you to fill in the blanks with your own personal ideas and information. If you like to write, you may want to fill in all the blanks. If you don't like to write, you can have someone write the answers for you or you can just discuss the answers. We all learn differently and need different levels of help.

There are three sections of the *Skills System Workbook*:

- *Pre-Learning:* These activities prepare you to learn skills and reach your goals.
- *Learning Skills:* The handouts, worked examples, and worksheets in this section teach skills concepts that you will use in your Skills Plans.
- *Reaching Goals:* These activities help you create Skills Plans that help you reach your goals.

WHAT YOU WILL LEARN

The Skills System is a set of nine skills that help us manage our feelings and reach our goals. This Workbook helps us learn skills and bring them into our daily lives. Skills support us to manage life, get what we need, and be who we want to be.

We begin the journey by exploring our goals. Getting to know ourselves and what we want helps us use skills to reach goals and live aligned with our values. Knowing what is important to us helps us be motivated to use skills and to try new things.

Once we are ready to start building our toolbox, we jump into the Learning Skills handouts, worksheets, and worked examples. Handouts teach skills concepts. Worksheets help us to apply the concepts in our lives. Worked examples show us how to complete worksheets and offer a sample of how concepts can be used. The worked examples in the Learning Skills section are for adults. There is a set of worked examples for elementary school-age children and high school-age youth available on this book's companion website (*www.guilford.com/brown14-materials*).

As we are learning skills, we can begin using the Reaching Goals worked examples and worksheets. We create Skills Plans, monitor our progress using skills, assess skills gaps, and make new, more effective Skills Plans. The *Skills System Workbook* gives us learning opportunities that help us increase our abilities to manage the ups and downs of life, while staying on-track to our goals.

Pre-Learning

If you would like to work on reaching specific goals in your life, I would recommend completing the Pre-Learning worked examples and worksheets. These topics will create a journey that helps you:

- Get to know yourself and your feelings in a deeper way.
- Focus on what actions you believe are working (and not working) in your current life.
- Clarify goals that are important to you.
- Highlight what actions to increase (or decrease) to help you reach your goals.

When we know what is important to us, we can create Skills Plans that both reflect our values and personality, and help us get what we want and need.

We are all evolving and learning each day! The information in the Pre-Learning worksheets is likely to change over time. Consider using a pencil to write in your answers so you can change and update them as you learn more about yourself and the skills. The ebook version of the *Skills System Workbook* allows you to type in answers (and change them whenever you need to), which can be helpful.

| PRE-LEARNING | WORKED EXAMPLE 1 |

Getting to Know Me

Name: _____   Date: _____

Directions: We are all changing and developing all the time. This worksheet is designed to help you get to know different parts of yourself. Remembering our strengths, supports, spirituality, and successes can help us manage challenges we face. Please list things that fit in each of the five areas below.

My Strengths _I am good at video games._
_____ _I think I am friendly._
_____ _I am good at basketball._

My Supports _My sister and I are close._
_____ _I have a best friend._
_____

My Spirituality _I used to go to church when I was younger._
_____
_____

My Challenges _I don't like where I live._
_____ _People tell me what to do a lot._
_____ _I want to get a job._

My Successes _I beat a lot of video games._
_____ _I have my own cell phone._
_____ _I had a girlfriend last year._

From *The Emotion Regulation Skills System Workbook, Second Edition.* Copyright © 2026 Julie F. Brown. Published by The Guilford Press. Permission to photocopy this material or download it from the epdf is granted to purchasers of this book for personal use; see copyright page for details.

PRE-LEARNING — **WORKSHEET 1**

Getting to Know Me

Name: _____ Date: _____

Directions: We are all changing and developing all the time. This worksheet is designed to help you get to know different parts of yourself. Remembering our strengths, supports, spirituality, and successes can help us manage challenges we face. Please list things that fit in each of the five areas below.

My Strengths _____

_____

_____

My Supports _____

_____

_____

My Spirituality _____

_____

_____

My Challenges _____

_____

_____

My Successes _____

_____

_____

From *The Emotion Regulation Skills System Workbook, Second Edition*. Copyright © 2026 Julie F. Brown. Published by The Guilford Press. Permission to photocopy this material or download it from the epdf is granted to purchasers of this book for personal use; see copyright page for details.

| PRE-LEARNING | WORKED EXAMPLE 2 |

Getting to Know My Feelings

Name: _____   Date: _____

Directions: Please read each of the six statements below. Check off the "Yes" box if you think the statement is true about your feelings. Check the "No" box if it does not describe your feelings. Check "Not Sure" if you are not sure. Add any description below the boxes to better explain your feelings.

I am a very sensitive person.

    ☒ Yes, I am.   ☐ No, not really.   ☐ Not sure

Describe: _I have a big heart. I cry a lot at the movies._

My feelings get strong, very quickly.

    ☒ Yes, they do.   ☐ No, they don't.   ☐ Not sure

Describe: _I get really mad, really fast._

It takes a long time for my feelings to come down.

    ☒ Yes, it does.   ☐ No, it doesn't.   ☐ Not sure

Describe: _I do stay upset for a really long time._

I sometimes act really quickly when I have feelings.

    ☒ Yes, I do.   ☐ No, I do not.   ☐ Not sure

Describe: _____

My feelings get in the way of me reaching my goals.

    ☒ Yes, they do.   ☐ No, they don't   ☐ Not sure

Describe: _I'm trying to get a full-time job, but I have a hard time keeping a part-time job._

From *The Emotion Regulation Skills System Workbook, Second Edition*. Copyright © 2026 Julie F. Brown. Published by The Guilford Press. Permission to photocopy this material or download it from the epdf is granted to purchasers of this book for personal use; see copyright page for details.

| PRE-LEARNING | WORKSHEET 2 |

Getting to Know My Feelings

Name: _____ Date: _____

Directions: Please read each of the six statements below. Check off the "Yes" box if you think the statement is true about your feelings. Check the "No" box if it does not describe your feelings. Check "Not Sure" if you are not sure. Add any description below the boxes to better explain your feelings.

I am a very sensitive person.

☐ Yes, I am.   ☐ No, not really.   ☐ Not sure

Describe: _____

My feelings get strong, very quickly.

☐ Yes, they do.   ☐ No, they don't.   ☐ Not sure

Describe: _____

It takes a long time for my feelings to come down.

☐ Yes, it does.   ☐ No, it doesn't.   ☐ Not sure

Describe: _____

I sometimes act really quickly when I have feelings.

☐ Yes, I do.   ☐ No, I do not.   ☐ Not sure

Describe: _____

My feelings get in the way of me reaching my goals.

☐ Yes, they do.   ☐ No, they don't   ☐ Not sure

Describe: _____

From *The Emotion Regulation Skills System Workbook, Second Edition*. Copyright © 2026 Julie F. Brown. Published by The Guilford Press. Permission to photocopy this material or download it from the epdf is granted to purchasers of this book for personal use; see copyright page for details.

| PRE-LEARNING | WORKED EXAMPLE 3 |

My New-Me and My Old-Me

Name: _____   Date: _____

Directions: List things under My New-Me that represent how you would like to be and things you would like in your life when you are on-track to your goals. Under My Old-Me list things that you do when you are off-track from your goals.

My New-Me

Live on my own.

Not yelling, hitting, and breaking stuff.

See my family more.

Have a girlfriend.

Get a job and make money.

Take my medications.

Have fun.

My Old-Me

Yelling at people when I'm mad.

Breaking things when I'm upset.

Not doing my chores.

Not taking my medications.

Wearing dirty clothes.

Hitting people.

From *The Emotion Regulation Skills System Workbook, Second Edition*. Copyright © 2026 Julie F. Brown. Published by The Guilford Press. Permission to photocopy this material or download it from the epdf is granted to purchasers of this book for personal use; see copyright page for details.

PRE-LEARNING **WORKSHEET 3**

My New-Me and My Old-Me

Name: _____   Date: _____

Directions: List things under My New-Me that represent how you would like to be and things you would like in your life when you are on-track to your goals. Under My Old-Me list things that you do when you are off-track from your goals.

My New-Me

_____
_____
_____
_____
_____
_____
_____

My Old-Me

_____
_____
_____
_____
_____
_____
_____

From *The Emotion Regulation Skills System Workbook, Second Edition*. Copyright © 2026 Julie F. Brown. Published by The Guilford Press. Permission to photocopy this material or download it from the epdf is granted to purchasers of this book for personal use; see copyright page for details.

| PRE-LEARNING | WORKED EXAMPLE 4 |

My Goals

Name: _____   Date: _____

Directions: Write down any goals you have. Some goals may be more important to you than others. After you write down all the goals, think about how important each of them is to you. Circle A, B, or C. An "A" goal is most important, "B" is very important, and "C" is important to you. Our goals can change, so add new goals and change or remove goals as you want to.

My Goal
I want to live in my own apartment.

Priority Level:
(A) = Most important
B = Very important
C = Important

My Goal
I want to get a job.

Priority Level:
A = Most important
(B) = Very important
C = Important

My Goal
I want to see my family more.

Priority Level:
A = Most important
(B) = Very important
C = Important

My Goal
I want to have a girlfriend.

Priority Level:
A = Most important
(B) = Very important
C = Important

My Goal
I want to join a basketball team.

Priority Level:
A = Most important
B = Very important
(C) = Important

My Goal
I want to get a dog.

Priority Level:
A = Most important
B = Very important
(C) = Important

From *The Emotion Regulation Skills System Workbook, Second Edition*. Copyright © 2026 Julie F. Brown. Published by The Guilford Press. Permission to photocopy this material or download it from the epdf is granted to purchasers of this book for personal use; see copyright page for details.

| PRE-LEARNING | WORKSHEET 4 |

My Goals

Name: _____ Date: _____

Directions: Write down any goals you have. Some goals may be more important to you than others. After you write down all the goals, think about how important each of them is to you. Circle A, B, or C. An "A" goal is most important, "B" is very important, and "C" is important to you. Our goals can change, so add new goals and change or remove goals as you want to.

My Goal
_____

Priority Level:
A = Most important
B = Very important
C = Important

My Goal
_____

Priority Level:
A = Most important
B = Very important
C = Important

My Goal
_____

Priority Level:
A = Most important
B = Very important
C = Important

My Goal
_____

Priority Level:
A = Most important
B = Very important
C = Important

My Goal
_____

Priority Level:
A = Most important
B = Very important
C = Important

My Goal
_____

Priority Level:
A = Most important
B = Very important
C = Important

From *The Emotion Regulation Skills System Workbook, Second Edition*. Copyright © 2026 Julie F. Brown. Published by The Guilford Press. Permission to photocopy this material or download it from the epdf is granted to purchasers of this book for personal use; see copyright page for details.

| PRE-LEARNING | WORKED EXAMPLE 5 |

Exploring My Goals

Name: _____   Date: _____

Directions: This worksheet is a chance to think about your life—how it is now and how you might like it to be. Filling in the answers to the following questions may help you set a personal goal. Complete one of these worksheets for each of the different things that you want to change in your life.

What do I want to change?
_____ *I don't want to live here.* _____

What is my current situation?
_____ *I live in a group home.* _____

How do I want my situation to be?
_____ *I want to have my own place without staff.* _____

Why is this important to me?
_____ *I don't like people telling me what to do.* _____

🏃 **What is My Goal?**
_____ *I want to live in an apartment.* _____

🚫 **What are barriers to My Goal?**

I don't have enough money.   *People won't help me move.*

I don't have a place to go.   *They say I'm not ready.*

From *The Emotion Regulation Skills System Workbook, Second Edition.* Copyright © 2026 Julie F. Brown. Published by The Guilford Press. Permission to photocopy this material or download it from the epdf is granted to purchasers of this book for personal use; see copyright page for details.

| PRE-LEARNING | WORKSHEET 5 |

Exploring My Goals

Name: _____   Date: _____

Directions: This worksheet is a chance to think about your life—how it is now and how you might like it to be. Filling in the answers to the following questions may help you set a personal goal. Complete one of these worksheets for each of the different things that you want to change in your life.

What do I want to change?
_____

What is my current situation?
_____

How do I want my situation to be?
_____

Why is this important to me?
_____

What is My Goal?
_____

What are barriers to My Goal?

_____   _____

_____   _____

From *The Emotion Regulation Skills System Workbook, Second Edition*. Copyright © 2026 Julie F. Brown. Published by The Guilford Press. Permission to photocopy this material or download it from the epdf is granted to purchasers of this book for personal use; see copyright page for details.

| PRE-LEARNING | WORKED EXAMPLE 6 |

Exploring Targets to Reach My Goal

Name: _____ Date: _____

Directions: Write one of your My Goals on the top line. Then list things you want or need to do MORE of and LESS of to reach My Goal.

My Goal: <u>I want to live in my own apartment.</u>

My Targets: Do MORE of
What do I want or need to do MORE of in my life to reach My Goal?

<u>Get a job so I can pay bills.</u>
<u>Get along with my housemate so I can leave here.</u>
<u>Do laundry and chores.</u>
<u>Take my medications like I am supposed to.</u>

My Targets: Do LESS of
What do I want or need to do LESS of in my life to reach My Goal?

<u>Stop yelling at people.</u>
<u>Don't skip my medications.</u>
<u>Stop hitting people.</u>

From *The Emotion Regulation Skills System Workbook, Second Edition.* Copyright © 2026 Julie F. Brown. Published by The Guilford Press. Permission to photocopy this material or download it from the epdf is granted to purchasers of this book for personal use; see copyright page for details.

| PRE-LEARNING | WORKSHEET 6 |

Exploring Targets to Reach My Goal

Name: _____   Date: _____

Directions: Write one of your My Goals on the top line. Then list things you want or need to do MORE of and LESS of to reach My Goal.

My Goal: _____

My Targets: Do MORE of

What do I want or need to do MORE of in my life to reach My Goal?

_____
_____
_____
_____
_____

My Targets: Do LESS of

What do I want or need to do LESS of in my life to reach My Goal?

_____
_____
_____
_____
_____

From *The Emotion Regulation Skills System Workbook, Second Edition*. Copyright © 2026 Julie F. Brown. Published by The Guilford Press. Permission to photocopy this material or download it from the epdf is granted to purchasers of this book for personal use; see copyright page for details.

Are You Ready to Learn Skills?

I know it can be difficult to start a new journey. You might have had feelings and experiences in the past that make learning skills seem scary or even impossible. You might not see yourself as a great learner. Maybe you hated school. You might have learned different skills that didn't work well or were hard to remember and use. All this can feel true AND you can still move ahead toward learning skills.

Here is some On-Track Thinking that can help you learn skills:

1. This workbook will guide me step by step.
2. I can go at my own pace.
3. I can learn in any way that fits me.
4. I can share this with others who can help me.
5. Learning skills will help me have a fuller toolbox of strategies to handle feelings.
6. Skills can help me reach my goals.
7. I can do this!

Enjoy and have fun!

Learning Skills

This section of the *Skills System Workbook* is broken down into 12 different parts.

1. Skills List
2. System Tools (i.e., Feelings Rating Scale, Categories of Skills, and Recipe for Skills)
3. Clear Picture
4. On-Track Thinking
5. On-Track Action
6. Safety Plan
7. New-Me Activities
8. Problem Solving
9. Expressing Myself
10. Getting It Right
11. Relationship Care
12. Using Skills in My Life

The first part introduces the nine core skills. Learning the names, numbers, and pictures that correspond to each skill is helpful! The second part explains the System Tools, which will help you put your Skills Plans together. Parts 3–11 provide in-depth teaching about the nine core skills in the Skills System. The final part focuses on reviewing skills concepts and practicing using skills in your daily lives.

Skills List

| LEARNING SKILLS, SKILLS LIST | HANDOUT 1 |

Directions: Below are the nine core skills in the Skills System. It is helpful to learn their names, numbers, and pictures.

Nine Core Skills

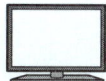 1. Clear Picture

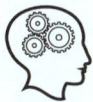 2. On-Track Thinking

 3. On-Track Action

 4. Safety Plan

 5. New-Me Activities

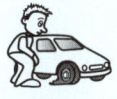 6. Problem Solving

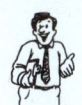 7. Expressing Myself

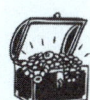 8. Getting It Right

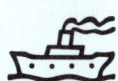 9. Relationship Care

From *The Emotion Regulation Skills System Workbook, Second Edition*. Copyright © 2026 Julie F. Brown. Published by The Guilford Press. Permission to photocopy this material or download it from the epdf is granted to purchasers of this book for personal use; see copyright page for details.

LEARNING SKILLS, SKILLS LIST   **HANDOUT 2**

How Our Skills Help Us

There are NINE skills in the Skills System.

Here is a list of the nine skills and how they help us. Knowing what skills do for us can help us know when and how to use skills in our lives.

All-the-Time Skills

 1. **Clear Picture:** Clear Picture helps me notice what is happening inside and outside of me *right now*. I see the situation as it is.

 2. **On-Track Thinking:** On-Track Thinking helps me think clearly about what I want and what will work to help me reach my goals.

 3. **On-Track Action:** Once I get a Clear Picture and have On-Track Thinking, I take an On-Track Action to do something to move toward my goals.

 4. **Safety Plan:** I use a Safety Plan to handle risky situations that are happening right now or may happen in the future.

 5. **New-Me Activities:** I do New-Me Activities to help me focus my attention, feel better, distract me, and have fun.

Calm-Only Skills

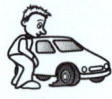 6. **Problem Solving:** I take time to solve problems in my life, so that I can be happier and reach my goals.

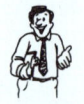 7. **Expressing Myself:** I share what is on my mind and in my heart to help me stay on-track with myself and other people.

 8. **Getting It Right:** Getting It Right helps me work with people to get what I want.

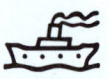 9. **RelationSHIP Care:** Relationship Care helps me understand how to have on-track relationships with myself and others.

From *The Emotion Regulation Skills System Workbook, Second Edition.* Copyright © 2026 Julie F. Brown. Published by The Guilford Press. Permission to photocopy this material or download it from the epdf is granted to purchasers of this book for personal use; see copyright page for details.

LEARNING SKILLS, SKILLS LIST   WORKSHEET 1

Name the Skill by Picture

Name: _____   Date: _____

Please fill in the name of each skill.

1. _____

2. _____

3. _____

4. _____

5. _____

6. _____

7. _____

8. _____

9. _____

From *The Emotion Regulation Skills System Workbook, Second Edition*. Copyright © 2026 Julie F. Brown. Published by The Guilford Press. Permission to photocopy this material or download it from the epdf is granted to purchasers of this book for personal use; see copyright page for details.

LEARNING SKILLS, SKILLS LIST

WORKSHEET 2

Match the Skill Number and Initials to the Picture

Name: _____ Date: _____

Please draw a line from the number of the skill to the correct picture.

1. **CP**

2. **OTT**

3. **OTA**

4. **SP**

5. **NMA**

6. **PS**

7. **EM**

8. **GIR**

9. **RC**

From *The Emotion Regulation Skills System Workbook, Second Edition.* Copyright © 2026 Julie F. Brown. Published by The Guilford Press. Permission to photocopy this material or download it from the epdf is granted to purchasers of this book for personal use; see copyright page for details.

LEARNING SKILLS, SKILLS LIST   **WORKSHEET 3**

Name the Skill by Number

Name: _____ Date: _____

Please fill in the name of each skill.

1. _____

2. _____

3. _____

4. _____

5. _____

6. _____

7. _____

8. _____

9. _____

From *The Emotion Regulation Skills System Workbook, Second Edition*. Copyright © 2026 Julie F. Brown. Published by The Guilford Press. Permission to photocopy this material or download it from the epdf is granted to purchasers of this book for personal use; see copyright page for details.

System Tools

| LEARNING SKILLS, SYSTEM TOOLS | HANDOUT 1 |

How I Use the Skills System

A. The Feelings Rating Scale

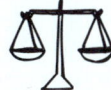

The Feelings Rating Scale is a 0–1–2–3–4–5 scale I use to rate how strong my feelings are. The Feelings Rating Scale helps me know what skills and how many skills I link together in a Skills Plan to manage a situation.

B. Categories of Skills

 All-the-Time 0–5 Emotion   **Calm-Only 0–3 Emotion**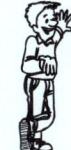

There are two Categories of Skills: All-the-Time skills and Calm-Only skills. I can use All-the-Time skills at any level of feeling: 0–1–2–3–4–5. I can only use Calm-Only skills when I am at a 0–1–2–3 feeling.

C. Recipe for Skills

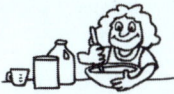

The Recipe for Skills helps me know the minimum number of skills I need to link together in a Skills Plan or Skills Chain. The recipe tells me to add one skill for every level of feeling (including 0). So, if I am at a 3 sad, I need to use at least four skills.

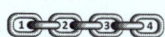

From *The Emotion Regulation Skills System Workbook, Second Edition.* Copyright © 2026 Julie F. Brown. Published by The Guilford Press. Permission to photocopy this material or download it from the epdf is granted to purchasers of this book for personal use; see copyright page for details.

LEARNING SKILLS, SYSTEM TOOLS

HANDOUT 2

Feelings Rating Scale with Pictures

At a 5, I harm myself, others, or property.

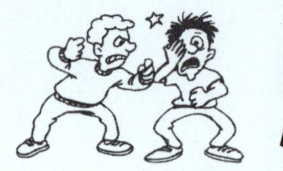

5

OVERWHELMING FEELING

At a 4, I have a hard time talking and listening and staying on-track.

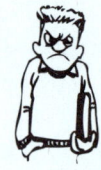

4

STRONG FEELING

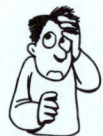

3

Medium feeling

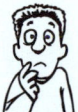

2

Small feeling

At 0–3 feelings, I can talk and listen and stay on-track.

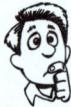

1

Tiny feeling

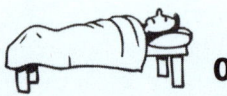

0

No feeling

From *The Emotion Regulation Skills System Workbook, Second Edition*. Copyright © 2026 Julie F. Brown. Published by The Guilford Press. Permission to photocopy this material or download it from the epdf is granted to purchasers of this book for personal use; see copyright page for details.

LEARNING SKILLS, SYSTEM TOOLS

HANDOUT 3

Feelings Rating Scale with Descriptions

Rating feelings using the 0–1–2–3–4–5 scale helps me to know which skills I should use AND how many skills I need to use.

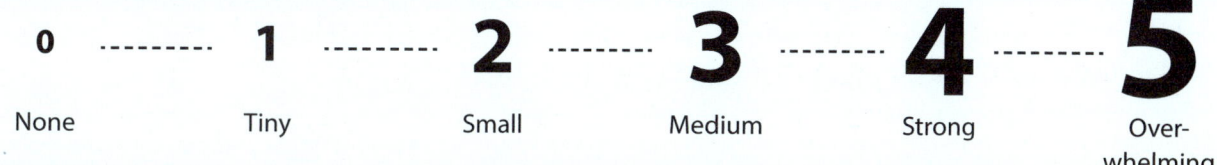

0	1	2	3	4	5
None	Tiny	Small	Medium	Strong	Over-whelming

Rating level	How I feel at different levels of feelings
0	A 0 is when I am not noticing a feeling. For example, a 0 anger means that I am not feeling angry at that moment. I can be a 2 sad and 0 angry.
1	A 1 is when I am having a tiny feeling. At a 1, I may notice just enough body sensations to label the feeling. The situation may make me feel a 1 or it may mean that a stronger feeling is beginning to happen. It may also mean that a stronger feeling is reducing to a 1. In all of these cases, at a 1, I am able to think clearly and control my urges, impulses, and actions. Because I am able to think clearly when I am at a 1 feeling, I can use all of my skills, even the Calm-Only ones! Because Expressing Myself increases feelings, it may be helpful to begin expressing at a Level 2 rather than a 3.
2	A 2 is when I am having a small feeling. I may notice more body sensations than at a Level 1. My thinking may be affected by the Level 2 reaction. For example, at a 2 angry, I may feel my heart beating faster and my thoughts may speed up. I am still able to think clearly, so I can use all of my skills at a 2, even the Calm-Only ones. This may be a good time to use Expressing Myself rather than at a 3 feeling or above.
3	A 3 is a medium feeling. This level of reaction will cause stronger body sensations. At a 3, these body sensations may make me feel uncomfortable. For example, at a 3 angry, my heart might pound and my breathing may be heavier. I can focus, talk, listen, and stay on-track, even though I am stressed. I can still use my Calm-Only skills at a 3 feeling. If I am unable to focus, stop listening, or raise my voice, I am going over a 3. I create problems for myself when I try to use Calm-Only skills over a 3.
4	A 4 is a strong feeling. At a 4 there will be strong body sensations, and it will be harder to control my thinking. When I notice I am at a Level 4, I can use all five of my All-the-Time skills to help me become calmer. If I don't use enough of the All-the-Time skills at a Level 4, I may try to use Expressing Myself and yell or do Problem Solving and make things worse! I have to wait to use my Calm-Only skills until I have gone down to or below a 3. I know I am at a 4 (rather than a 5) when I have strong feelings but do not hurt myself, others, or property.
5	A 5 is an overwhelming feeling. At a 5, I am not in control. The body sensations, thoughts, and urges are overwhelming. At a 5, I take actions that hurt myself, others, or property. For example, at a 5 anger, I may break a window on purpose. My emotional mind is in the driver's seat (rather than my skills) and I do things that I regret. I have to use *all* of my All-the-Time skills and double up on New-Me Activities or On-Track Actions to get back on-track.

From *The Emotion Regulation Skills System Workbook, Second Edition*. Copyright © 2026 Julie F. Brown. Published by The Guilford Press. Permission to photocopy this material or download it from the epdf is granted to purchasers of this book for personal use; see copyright page for details.

LEARNING SKILLS, SYSTEM TOOLS | **WORKED EXAMPLE 1**

Feelings Rating Scale

Name: _____   Date: _____

Please list events and feelings for each level 0–5.

I blink my eyes.
_____   **0**   Anger
When this happens, I don't feel.   No feeling

My stomach growls.
_____   **1**   Hungry
When this happens, I feel →   Tiny feeling

There is no good food in the house.
_____   **2**   Frustrated
When this happens, I feel →   Small feeling

I order a pizza to be delivered.
_____   **3**   Excited
When this happens, I feel →   Medium feeling

The pizza man yells at me and I feel frozen.
_____   **4**   Nervous
When this happens, I feel →   Strong feeling

I drop the pizza and slam the door.
_____   **5**   Fear
When this happens, I feel →   Overwhelming feeling

From *The Emotion Regulation Skills System Workbook, Second Edition*. Copyright © 2026 Julie F. Brown. Published by The Guilford Press. Permission to photocopy this material or download it from the epdf is granted to purchasers of this book for personal use; see copyright page for details.

LEARNING SKILLS, SYSTEM TOOLS **WORKSHEET 1**

Feelings Rating Scale

Name: _____ Date: _____

Please list events and feelings for each level 0–5.

_____ **0** _____

When this happens, I don't feel. No feeling

_____ **1** _____

When this happens, I feel → Tiny feeling

_____ **2** _____

When this happens, I feel → Small feeling

_____ **3** _____

When this happens, I feel → Medium feeling

_____ **4** _____

When this happens, I feel → Strong feeling

_____ **5** _____

When this happens, I feel → Over-whelming feeling

From *The Emotion Regulation Skills System Workbook, Second Edition*. Copyright © 2026 Julie F. Brown. Published by The Guilford Press. Permission to photocopy this material or download it from the epdf is granted to purchasers of this book for personal use; see copyright page for details.

LEARNING SKILLS, SYSTEM TOOLS HANDOUT 4

Categories of Skills

Once I know my level of feeling (0–1–2–3–4–5), I know what Category of Skills I can use:

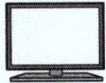 1. Clear Picture

 2. On-Track Thinking

 3. On-Track Action

 4. Safety Plan

 5. New-Me Activities

All-the-Time skills

0–5 feelings

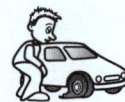 6. Problem Solving

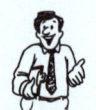 7. Expressing Myself

 8. Getting It Right

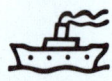 9. Relationship Care

Calm-Only skills

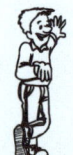

Only 0–3 feelings!

From *The Emotion Regulation Skills System Workbook, Second Edition.* Copyright © 2026 Julie F. Brown. Published by The Guilford Press. Permission to photocopy this material or download it from the epdf is granted to purchasers of this book for personal use; see copyright page for details.

| LEARNING SKILLS, SYSTEM TOOLS | WORKSHEET 2 |

Name the Skills and Categories of Skills

Name: _____ Date: _____

Please fill in the Skills List and Categories of Skills.

📺 _____

🧠 _____

🚂 _____   _____

🛡️ _____   _____

☕ _____

0–1–2–3–4–5

🚗 _____

👔 _____   _____

💰 _____   _____

🚢 _____

0–1–2–3

From *The Emotion Regulation Skills System Workbook, Second Edition*. Copyright © 2026 Julie F. Brown. Published by The Guilford Press. Permission to photocopy this material or download it from the epdf is granted to purchasers of this book for personal use; see copyright page for details.

LEARNING SKILLS, SYSTEM TOOLS　　　　　　　**WORKED EXAMPLE 2**

Select the Category of Skills by Feelings Level

Name: _____   Date: _____

Please circle the skills that can be used when you are having these feelings.

Level	Feeling		
3	Frustrated	(All-the-Time skills)	Calm-Only skills
5	Anger	All-the-Time skills	Calm-Only skills
4	Scared	All-the-Time skills	Calm-Only skills
2	Joy	All-the-Time skills	(Calm-Only skills)
4½	Sad	All-the-Time skills	Calm-Only skills
1	Envy	All-the-Time skills	(Calm-Only skills)
3	Happiness	All-the-Time skills	(Calm-Only skills)
3½	Shame	(All-the-Time skills)	Calm-Only skills

From *The Emotion Regulation Skills System Workbook, Second Edition*. Copyright © 2026 Julie F. Brown. Published by The Guilford Press. Permission to photocopy this material or download it from the epdf is granted to purchasers of this book for personal use; see copyright page for details.

LEARNING SKILLS, SYSTEM TOOLS **WORKSHEET 3**

Select the Category of Skills by Feelings Level

Name: _____   Date: _____

Please circle the skills that can be used when you are having these feelings.

3	Sad	All-the-Time skills	Calm-Only skills
5	Fear	All-the-Time skills	Calm-Only skills
4	Disgusted	All-the-Time skills	Calm-Only skills
2	Happy	All-the-Time skills	Calm-Only skills
4½	Jealous	All-the-Time skills	Calm-Only skills
1	Mad	All-the-Time skills	Calm-Only skills
3	Love	All-the-Time skills	Calm-Only skills
3½	Guilty	All-the-Time skills	Calm-Only skills

From *The Emotion Regulation Skills System Workbook, Second Edition*. Copyright © 2026 Julie F. Brown. Published by The Guilford Press. Permission to photocopy this material or download it from the epdf is granted to purchasers of this book for personal use; see copyright page for details.

| LEARNING SKILLS, SYSTEM TOOLS | WORKSHEET 4 |

Feelings Ratings and Categories of Skills

Name: _____ Date: _____

Please write feelings and rating levels in the blanks. Then circle the skills that can be used when at those levels.

Rating and Feeling

_____ _____   🕘 All-the-Time skills   🧍 Calm-Only skills

_____ _____   🕘 All-the-Time skills   🧍 Calm-Only skills

_____ _____   🕘 All-the-Time skills   🧍 Calm-Only skills

_____ _____   🕘 All-the-Time skills   🧍 Calm-Only skills

_____ _____   🕘 All-the-Time skills   🧍 Calm-Only skills

_____ _____   🕘 All-the-Time skills   🧍 Calm-Only skills

_____ _____   🕘 All-the-Time skills   🧍 Calm-Only skills

_____ _____   🕘 All-the-Time skills   🧍 Calm-Only skills

From *The Emotion Regulation Skills System Workbook, Second Edition.* Copyright © 2026 Julie F. Brown. Published by The Guilford Press. Permission to photocopy this material or download it from the epdf is granted to purchasers of this book for personal use; see copyright page for details.

LEARNING SKILLS, SYSTEM TOOLS — HANDOUT 5

Recipe for Skills

Once I know my level of feeling (0–1–2–3–4–5), I use the Recipe for Skills to decide how many skills I link together in a skills chain. Skills masters use more!

 **Combine one skill for EVERY level of feeling:**

Level 0 feeling = At least one skill

Level 1 feeling = At least two skills

Level 2 feeling = At least three skills

Level 3 feeling = At least four skills

Level 4 feeling = At least five skills

Level 5 feeling = At least six skills

Helpful Hints:

Bigger feelings need more skills in my Skills Plan.

Smaller feelings can pass in a few moments. Larger feelings are more intense and last longer. I use more skills one after another in skills chains to deal with larger feelings.

Double up on All-the-Time skills at a Level 5 feeling.

At a Level 5 feeling, I need six skills. If I can't use my Calm-Only skills over a 3, what is the sixth skill I use? I do more All-the-Time skills such as On-Track Actions and New-Me Activities.

From *The Emotion Regulation Skills System Workbook, Second Edition.* Copyright © 2026 Julie F. Brown. Published by The Guilford Press. Permission to photocopy this material or download it from the epdf is granted to purchasers of this book for personal use; see copyright page for details.

| LEARNING SKILLS, SYSTEM TOOLS | WORKED EXAMPLE 3 |

Recipe for Skills: Choose How Many Skills to Use

Name: _____ Date: _____

Please circle the minimum number of skills that should be linked at these levels.

_3_	Frustrated	1 2 3 ④ 5 6
_5_	Anger	1 2 3 4 5 ⑥
_4_	Scared	1 2 3 4 ⑤ 6
_2_	Joy	1 2 ③ 4 5 6
_4½_	Sad	1 2 3 4 5 ⑥
_1_	Envy	1 ② 3 4 5 6
_3_	Happiness	1 2 3 ④ 5 6
_3½_	Shame	1 2 3 4 ⑤ 6

From *The Emotion Regulation Skills System Workbook, Second Edition*. Copyright © 2026 Julie F. Brown. Published by The Guilford Press. Permission to photocopy this material or download it from the epdf is granted to purchasers of this book for personal use; see copyright page for details.

LEARNING SKILLS, SYSTEM TOOLS — **WORKSHEET 5**

Recipe for Skills: Choose How Many Skills to Use

Name: _____   Date: _____

Please circle the minimum number of skills that should be linked at these levels.

3	Sad	1	2	3	4	5	6
5	Fear	1	2	3	4	5	6
4	Disgusted	1	2	3	4	5	6
2	Happy	1	2	3	4	5	6
4½	Jealous	1	2	3	4	5	6
1	Mad	1	2	3	4	5	6
3	Love	1	2	3	4	5	6
3	Guilty	1	2	3	4	5	6

From *The Emotion Regulation Skills System Workbook, Second Edition*. Copyright © 2026 Julie F. Brown. Published by The Guilford Press. Permission to photocopy this material or download it from the epdf is granted to purchasers of this book for personal use; see copyright page for details.

LEARNING SKILLS, SYSTEM TOOLS — WORKSHEET 6

Build Your Recipe for Skills

Name: _____ Date: _____

Please write rating levels and labels for the feelings in the blanks (like 4 sad). Circle the number of skills you need to link together.

Rating and Feeling

____ _____   1   2   3   4   5   6

____ _____   1   2   3   4   5   6

____ _____   1   2   3   4   5   6

____ _____   1   2   3   4   5   6

____ _____   1   2   3   4   5   6

____ _____   1   2   3   4   5   6

____ _____   1   2   3   4   5   6

____ _____   1   2   3   4   5   6

From *The Emotion Regulation Skills System Workbook, Second Edition*. Copyright © 2026 Julie F. Brown. Published by The Guilford Press. Permission to photocopy this material or download it from the epdf is granted to purchasers of this book for personal use; see copyright page for details.

LEARNING SKILLS, SYSTEM TOOLS — WORKED EXAMPLE 4

Week 2 Practice Activity

Name: _____   Date: _____

Directions: Think of a challenging situation that happened recently. Answer the questions using the System Tools.

Briefly describe a situation when you felt stressed this week.

I heard my best friend lost her job.

Feelings Rating Scale:

I felt __Sad__ at a Level __2__.

Categories of Skills:

I use my All-the-Time skills when I am at a __0__ to a __5__ feeling.

Could I use my All-the-Time skills in the stressful situation?   (YES) or NO

I use my Calm-Only skills when I am at a __0__ to a __3__ feeling.

Could I use my Calm-Only skills?   (YES) or NO

Recipe for Skills:

I was at a __2__ feeling, so I needed to use __3__ skills.

From *The Emotion Regulation Skills System Workbook, Second Edition*. Copyright © 2026 Julie F. Brown. Published by The Guilford Press. Permission to photocopy this material or download it from the epdf is granted to purchasers of this book for personal use; see copyright page for details.

LEARNING SKILLS, SYSTEM TOOLS **WORKSHEET 7**

Week 2 Practice Activity

Name: _____   Date: _____

Directions: Think of a challenging situation that happened recently. Answer the questions using the System Tools.

Briefly describe a situation when you felt stressed this week.

_____

_____

Feelings Rating Scale:

I felt _____ at a Level _____.

Categories of Skills:

I use my All-the-Time skills when I am at a _____ to a _____ feeling.

Could I use my All-the-Time skills in the stressful situation?   YES or NO

I use my Calm-Only skills when I am at a _____ to a _____ feeling.

Could I use my Calm-Only skills?   YES or NO

Recipe for Skills:

I was at a _____ feeling, so I needed to use _____ skills.

From *The Emotion Regulation Skills System Workbook, Second Edition.* Copyright © 2026 Julie F. Brown. Published by The Guilford Press. Permission to photocopy this material or download it from the epdf is granted to purchasers of this book for personal use; see copyright page for details.

LEARNING SKILLS, SYSTEM TOOLS

Review Questions

1. What is Skill 1?

2. What is Skill 2?

3. What is Skill 3?

4. What is Skill 4?

5. What is Skill 5?

6. What is Skill 6?

7. What is Skill 7?

8. What is Skill 8?

9. What is Skill 9?

10. What is the Feelings Rating Scale?

11. What are the Categories of Skills?

12. Which skills are All-the-Time skills?

13. At what level of feeling can we use the All-the-Time skills?

14. Which skills are the Calm-Only skills?

15. At what level of feeling can we use the Calm-Only skills?

16. What is the Recipe for Skills?

17. What are the six Clear Picture Do's? (Add this question after completing Week 3 Clear Picture.)

From *The Emotion Regulation Skills System Workbook, Second Edition*. Copyright © 2026 Julie F. Brown. Published by The Guilford Press. Permission to photocopy this material or download it from the epdf is granted to purchasers of this book for personal use; see copyright page for details.

Clear Picture

LEARNING SKILLS, CLEAR PICTURE — SUMMARY SHEET

Getting a Clear Picture

Clear Picture is an All-the-Time skill. I use my Clear Picture skill at all levels of feeling, 0–1–2–3–4–5. When I notice my feelings or situation change, I take a moment to get a Clear Picture of what is happening inside and outside of me. I guide my attention to be mindful of the six different parts of this one moment.

1. I **Notice My Breath.** I notice the air going in and out. I notice my breath as it is. I can notice the coolness of the breath in my nose. I can also notice the air filling my chest and belly. Bringing my attention to the breath, focusing 100% on it, helps me to be aware of myself in my present moment. In the breath, I handle *this one moment*, which is easier than managing my past and future moments.

2. I **Check My Surroundings.** I notice what is going on around me using my senses (see, hear, smell, taste, and touch). I notice what is happening in the situation right now. Some things might be physical and other things might be intangible. Some things might comfort me and others might not. I may not like what is happening and I have to see it clearly to deal with it. When I focus on how things should be, rather accepting the moment as it is, my emotions can go up.

3. I do a **Body Check.** I notice my body sensations. Emotions and thoughts may cause body sensations. The different body sensations help me be mindful of how I am feeling. Body sensations come and go, even intense ones. I notice the sensations as they are.

4. I **Label and Rate** my feelings. I notice emotions such as joy, peace, happiness, sadness, fear, jealousy, guilt, and anger. I notice other feelings such as hunger, tiredness, and stress that affect my mood. I may have more than one emotion or feeling at one time. Once I label a feeling, I rate how strong it is, using my 0–1–2–3–4–5 scale. Feelings, both pleasant and uncomfortable ones, come and go. I allow the emotions to pass like clouds, without holding on to them or pushing them away.

5. I **Notice My Thoughts.** My brain is active and creates many thoughts all day long. Noticing thoughts in my mind is like watching my thoughts moving across a TV screen. I notice some are automatic thoughts that pop into my mind. Others I create in my mind like self-talk. I watch all these thoughts come and go, like watching city buses pass by. Some thoughts are helpful; others are not. Some buses are going where I want to go and others do not. Just because I have a thought doesn't mean it is true; it is not who I am. I observe and accept thoughts in Clear Picture. Off-track thoughts can be challenging, but I remember that just because I notice a thought doesn't mean it is my plan. (I make plans in On-Track Thinking.)

6. I **Notice My Urges.** Urges make me feel like taking actions. Some of the urges are small; others are powerful. Urges can make me want to act on impulse. I have to remember that urges, like feelings and thoughts, come and go. This means that I can have powerful off-track urges and not take action on them. I don't ignore urges; instead I use Clear Picture and On-Track Thinking and take On-Track Actions to manage them.

From *The Emotion Regulation Skills System Workbook, Second Edition*. Copyright © 2026 Julie F. Brown. Published by The Guilford Press. Permission to photocopy this material or download it from the epdf is granted to purchasers of this book for personal use; see copyright page for details.

LEARNING SKILLS, CLEAR PICTURE HANDOUT 1

Clear Picture Do's

Focus 100% on the Clear Picture Do's to be aware of this one moment as it is.

1. Notice my breath

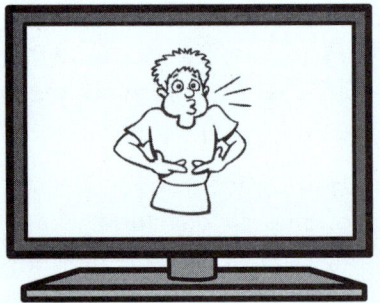

Where do I feel my breath?
What does it feel like?

2. Check my surroundings

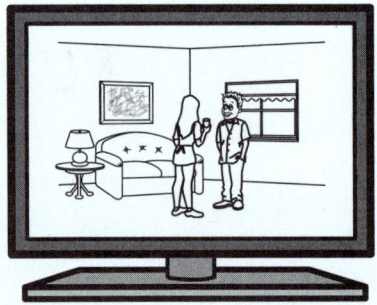

What is around me right now?
What do I see, hear, smell, taste, and touch?

3. Body check

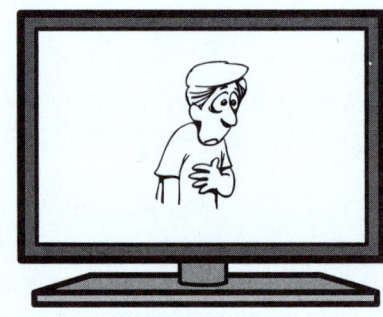

What body sensations do I feel right now?

4. Label and rate my feelings

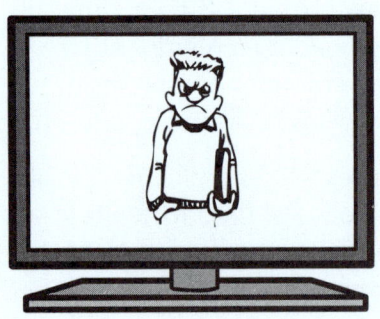

What feelings do I notice right now?
How strong are they?
0 1 2 3 4 5

5. Notice my thoughts

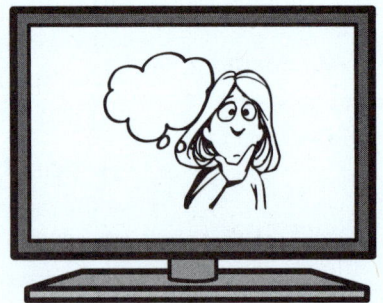

What thoughts do I notice going through my mind right now?

6. Notice my urges

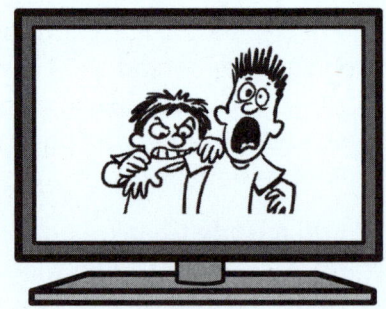

What do I feel like doing right now?

From *The Emotion Regulation Skills System Workbook, Second Edition.* Copyright © 2026 Julie F. Brown. Published by The Guilford Press. Permission to photocopy this material or download it from the epdf is granted to purchasers of this book for personal use; see copyright page for details.

LEARNING SKILLS, CLEAR PICTURE   **WORKED EXAMPLE 1**

Getting a Clear Picture

Name: _____   Date: _____

Get a clear picture: Please write what you are noticing in this one moment.

Situation: _I am opening the door on the first day of my new job._

Breath
I notice my breath is shallow.

Surroundings
The lights are on inside.
I don't see anyone I know.

Body Check
I have a pit in my stomach.
My heart is beating fast.

Feelings
I feel anxious at a Level 3.

Thoughts
I hope I like this job.

Urges
Go home.

From *The Emotion Regulation Skills System Workbook, Second Edition*. Copyright © 2026 Julie F. Brown. Published by The Guilford Press. Permission to photocopy this material or download it from the epdf is granted to purchasers of this book for personal use; see copyright page for details.

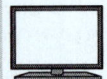 **LEARNING SKILLS, CLEAR PICTURE** **WORKSHEET 1**

Getting a Clear Picture

Name: _____ Date: _____

Get a clear picture: Please write what you are noticing in this one moment.

Situation: _____

Breath
_____
_____

Surroundings
_____
_____

Body Check
_____
_____

Feelings
_____
_____

Thoughts
_____
_____

Urges
_____
_____

From *The Emotion Regulation Skills System Workbook, Second Edition.* Copyright © 2026 Julie F. Brown. Published by The Guilford Press. Permission to photocopy this material or download it from the epdf is granted to purchasers of this book for personal use; see copyright page for details.

| LEARNING SKILLS, CLEAR PICTURE | WORKSHEET 2 |

Notice My Breath

Name: _____   Date: _____

I turn my attention to my breathing and notice it as it is.

Where do I notice my breath?

I can feel the air going in and out of my nose.

What does it feel like? _____

I can feel my chest rise and fall.

What does it feel like? _____

I bring the air in and out of my belly.

What does it feel like? _____

What do I notice about my breathing?

Is it shallow or deep?

What does it feel like? _____

Is it fast or slow?

What does it feel like? _____

From *The Emotion Regulation Skills System Workbook, Second Edition*. Copyright © 2026 Julie F. Brown. Published by The Guilford Press. Permission to photocopy this material or download it from the epdf is granted to purchasers of this book for personal use; see copyright page for details.

| LEARNING SKILLS, CLEAR PICTURE | HANDOUT 2 |

Notice Surroundings

I use my senses to get a Clear Picture of my surroundings.

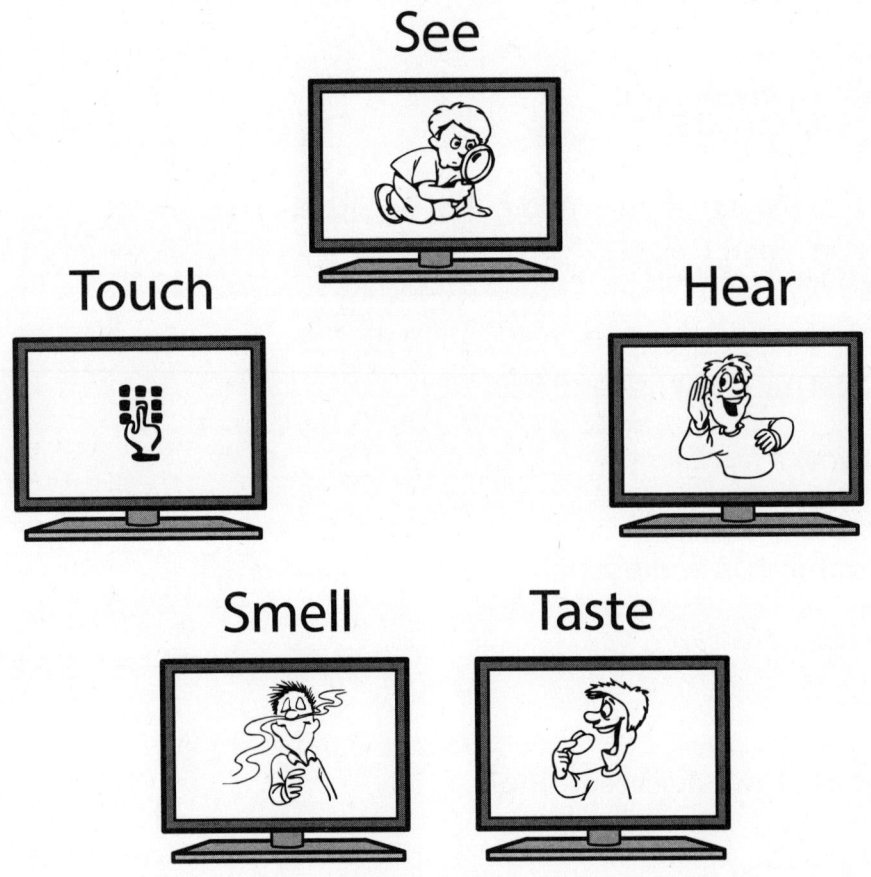

From *The Emotion Regulation Skills System Workbook, Second Edition*. Copyright © 2026 Julie F. Brown. Published by The Guilford Press. Permission to photocopy this material or download it from the epdf is granted to purchasers of this book for personal use; see copyright page for details.

LEARNING SKILLS, CLEAR PICTURE   **WORKED EXAMPLE 2**

Notice Surroundings

Name: _____ Date: _____

Please check your surroundings and write down what you notice.

Location: _I am sitting in my living room._____

I see _the TV, the furniture._____

I hear _the TV, a dog barking outside._____

I taste _the tea I am drinking._____

I smell _the lemon in my tea._____

I touch _the warm cup, the soft couch._____

From *The Emotion Regulation Skills System Workbook, Second Edition.* Copyright © 2026 Julie F. Brown. Published by The Guilford Press. Permission to photocopy this material or download it from the epdf is granted to purchasers of this book for personal use; see copyright page for details.

LEARNING SKILLS, CLEAR PICTURE WORKSHEET 3

Notice Surroundings

Name: _____   Date: _____

Please check your surroundings and write down what you notice.

Location: _____

I see _____

I hear _____

I taste _____

I smell _____

I touch _____

From *The Emotion Regulation Skills System Workbook, Second Edition.* Copyright © 2026 Julie F. Brown. Published by The Guilford Press. Permission to photocopy this material or download it from the epdf is granted to purchasers of this book for personal use; see copyright page for details.

| LEARNING SKILLS, CLEAR PICTURE | WORKED EXAMPLE 3 |

Body Check

Name: _____ Date: _____

What sensations do you feel in each part of your body?

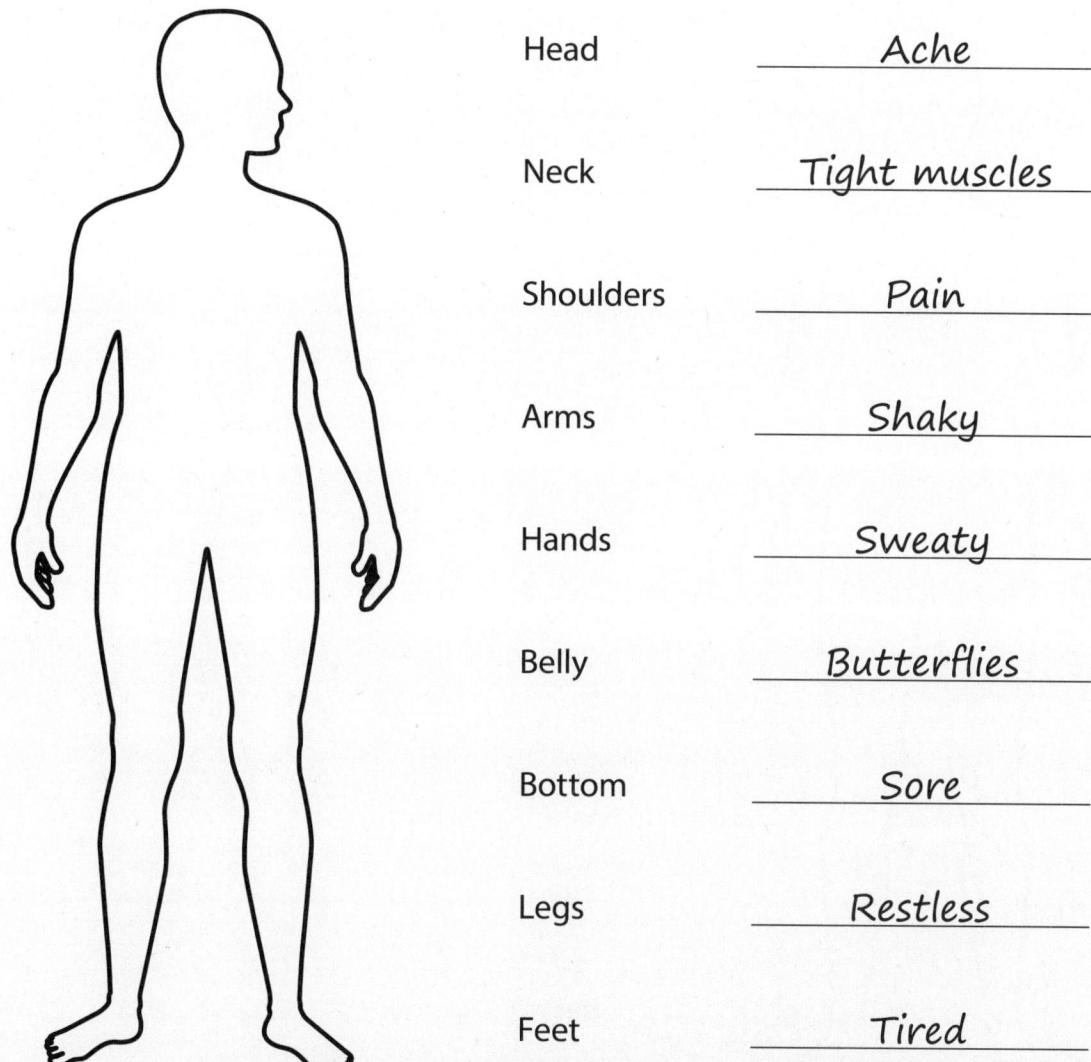

Head	Ache
Neck	Tight muscles
Shoulders	Pain
Arms	Shaky
Hands	Sweaty
Belly	Butterflies
Bottom	Sore
Legs	Restless
Feet	Tired

From *The Emotion Regulation Skills System Workbook, Second Edition*. Copyright © 2026 Julie F. Brown. Published by The Guilford Press. Permission to photocopy this material or download it from the epdf is granted to purchasers of this book for personal use; see copyright page for details.

LEARNING SKILLS, CLEAR PICTURE   **WORKSHEET 4**

Body Check

Name: _____   Date: _____

What sensations do you feel in each part of your body?

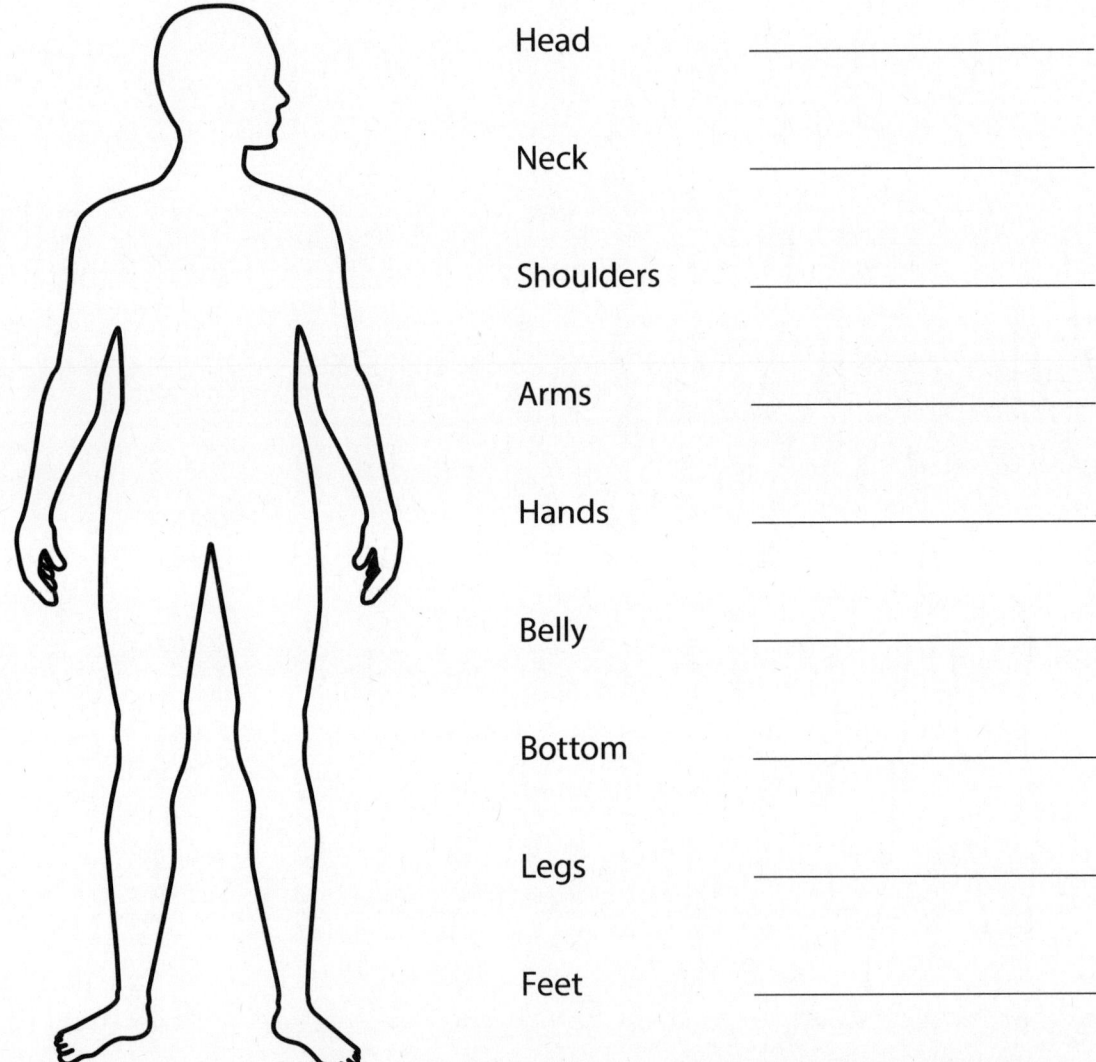

Head   _____

Neck   _____

Shoulders _____

Arms   _____

Hands   _____

Belly   _____

Bottom   _____

Legs   _____

Feet   _____

From *The Emotion Regulation Skills System Workbook, Second Edition*. Copyright © 2026 Julie F. Brown. Published by The Guilford Press. Permission to photocopy this material or download it from the epdf is granted to purchasers of this book for personal use; see copyright page for details.

LEARNING SKILLS, CLEAR PICTURE — **WORKED EXAMPLE 4**

Body Check: Sensations by Feelings Level

Name: _____   Date: _____

Please choose a feeling. List body sensations for each level of that feeling.

Feeling: _Anger_ _____

- **0** — I am smiling.
- **1** — I stop smiling, I squint my eyes a little.
- **2** — I tighten my lips, I make a frown.
- **3** — My jaw muscles tighten, my heart beats faster.
- **4** — My fists tighten, my chest is exploding inside.
- **5** — My mind and body feel like a tornado.

From *The Emotion Regulation Skills System Workbook, Second Edition*. Copyright © 2026 Julie F. Brown. Published by The Guilford Press. Permission to photocopy this material or download it from the epdf is granted to purchasers of this book for personal use; see copyright page for details.

LEARNING SKILLS, CLEAR PICTURE　　　　**WORKSHEET 5**

Body Check: Sensations by Feelings Level

Name: _____   Date: _____

Please choose a feeling. List body sensations for each level of that feeling.

Feeling: _____

0 _____

1 _____

2 _____

3 _____

4 _____

5 _____

From *The Emotion Regulation Skills System Workbook, Second Edition*. Copyright © 2026 Julie F. Brown. Published by The Guilford Press. Permission to photocopy this material or download it from the epdf is granted to purchasers of this book for personal use; see copyright page for details.

LEARNING SKILLS, CLEAR PICTURE   HANDOUT 3

Label and Rate Feelings: List of Feelings and Emotions

Please brainstorm a list of all possible emotions and feelings. A few examples are listed here. List all the other emotions and feelings you can think of.

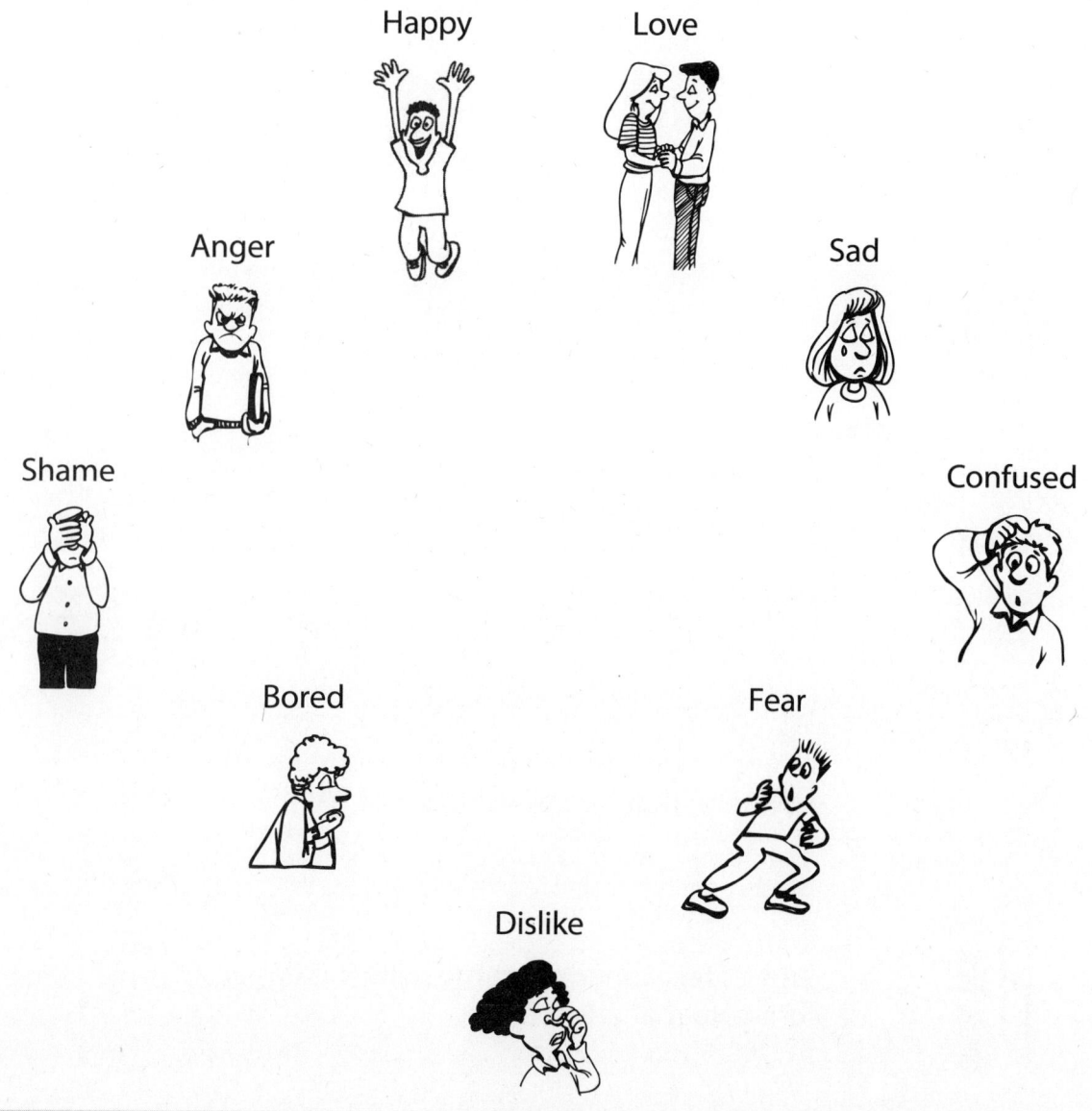

From *The Emotion Regulation Skills System Workbook, Second Edition*. Copyright © 2026 Julie F. Brown. Published by The Guilford Press. Permission to photocopy this material or download it from the epdf is granted to purchasers of this book for personal use; see copyright page for details.

LEARNING SKILLS, CLEAR PICTURE — HANDOUT 4

Label and Rate Feelings: How Feelings Affect Me

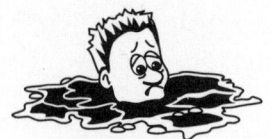 I react to situations with feelings.

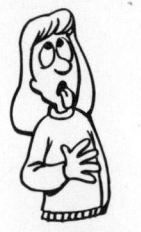 Feelings can affect how my body feels.

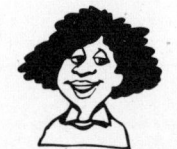 Feelings can affect how my face looks.

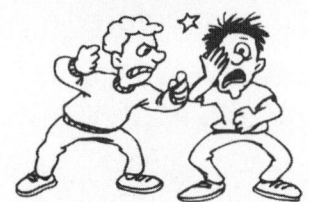 When I have feelings, I may want to take action.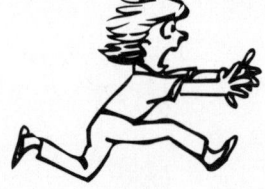

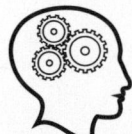 I can change how strong my feelings are and how long they last by using skills.

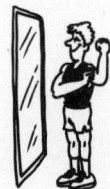 When I feel confident in my skills, it is easier for me to manage feelings.

From *The Emotion Regulation Skills System Workbook, Second Edition*. Copyright © 2026 Julie F. Brown. Published by The Guilford Press. Permission to photocopy this material or download it from the epdf is granted to purchasers of this book for personal use; see copyright page for details.

LEARNING SKILLS, CLEAR PICTURE — WORKED EXAMPLE 5

Label and Rate Feelings in Specific Situations

Name: _____ Date: _____

Please list situations when you might have each feeling.

Situation	Feeling	Rating
Going out to dinner with my friends	Happy	2
When I think about my best friend	Love	3
Thinking about family I miss	Sad	4
When my doctor told me about my medications	Confused	3
On the first day of a new job	Fear	2
When my boyfriend cheated on me	Dislike	4
When I have nothing to do	Bored	2
When I think about hurting people in the past	Shame	3
When someone steals my stuff	Anger	4

From *The Emotion Regulation Skills System Workbook, Second Edition*. Copyright © 2026 Julie F. Brown. Published by The Guilford Press. Permission to photocopy this material or download it from the epdf is granted to purchasers of this book for personal use; see copyright page for details.

LEARNING SKILLS, CLEAR PICTURE WORKSHEET 6

Label and Rate Feelings in Specific Situations

Name: _____   Date: _____

Please list situations when you might have each feeling.

	Feeling	Rating
_____	Happy	_____
_____	Love	_____
_____	Sad	_____
_____	Confused	_____
_____	Fear	_____
_____	Dislike	_____
_____	Bored	_____
_____	Shame	_____
_____	Anger	_____

From *The Emotion Regulation Skills System Workbook, Second Edition*. Copyright © 2026 Julie F. Brown. Published by The Guilford Press. Permission to photocopy this material or download it from the epdf is granted to purchasers of this book for personal use; see copyright page for details.

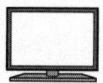 **LEARNING SKILLS, CLEAR PICTURE** HANDOUT 5

Noticing My Thoughts

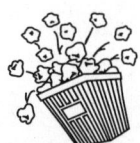

2. My mind makes lots of thoughts, like a popcorn machine. Some thoughts are helpful and others are not.

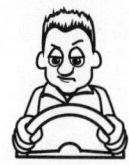

1. I turn my attention to my thoughts.

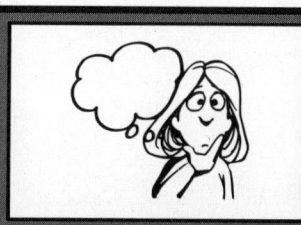

3. Thoughts go through my mind like city buses pass by on the street.

5. I can allow off-track thoughts to pass like a cloud through the sky.

4. Some will take me to my goal and some will not.

From *The Emotion Regulation Skills System Workbook, Second Edition*. Copyright © 2026 Julie F. Brown. Published by The Guilford Press. Permission to photocopy this material or download it from the epdf is granted to purchasers of this book for personal use; see copyright page for details.

LEARNING SKILLS, CLEAR PICTURE — **WORKED EXAMPLE 6**

Situations That Lead to Noticing Thoughts

Name: _____ Date: _____

Directions: Situations make us have thoughts. In Clear Picture we notice our thoughts as they pass through our mind. We don't change thoughts in Clear Picture—we just notice them. Write down a situation and a thought that you might have.

Situation: _____ I hit my toe really hard on my bed frame. _____
↘
Thought: _____

Situation: _____ The dog next door keeps barking. _____
↘
Thought: _____

Situation: _____ Someone is staring at me. _____
↘
Thought: _____

Situation: _____ I have a day off from work. _____
↘
Thought: _____

Situation: _____ It is my day to vacuum. _____
↘
Thought: _____

From *The Emotion Regulation Skills System Workbook, Second Edition*. Copyright © 2026 Julie F. Brown. Published by The Guilford Press. Permission to photocopy this material or download it from the epdf is granted to purchasers of this book for personal use; see copyright page for details.

| LEARNING SKILLS, CLEAR PICTURE | WORKSHEET 7 |

Situations That Lead to Noticing Thoughts

Name: _____   Date: _____

Directions: Situations make us have thoughts. In Clear Picture we notice our thoughts as they pass through our mind. We don't change thoughts in Clear Picture—we just notice them. Write down a situation and a thought that you might have.

Situation: _____
↘
   Thought: _____

Situation: _____
↘
   Thought: _____

Situation: _____
↘
   Thought: _____

Situation: _____
↘
   Thought: _____

Situation: _____
↘
   Thought: _____

From *The Emotion Regulation Skills System Workbook, Second Edition.* Copyright © 2026 Julie F. Brown. Published by The Guilford Press. Permission to photocopy this material or download it from the epdf is granted to purchasers of this book for personal use; see copyright page for details.

LEARNING SKILLS, CLEAR PICTURE WORKED EXAMPLE 7

Noticing Thoughts at Different Feelings Levels

Name: _____ Date: _____

Please list thoughts that may go with each feeling and level.

		Rating
I am doing a good job!	Happy	2
My brother is my best friend.	Love	3
I miss my family.	Sad	3
I don't know what I am doing.	Confused	2
That man is going to yell at me.	Fear	4
That woman was mean to me.	Dislike	4
I am sick of just watching TV.	Bored	1
I am ugly.	Shame	3
I hate how she looks at me.	Anger	4

From *The Emotion Regulation Skills System Workbook, Second Edition.* Copyright © 2026 Julie F. Brown. Published by The Guilford Press. Permission to photocopy this material or download it from the epdf is granted to purchasers of this book for personal use; see copyright page for details.

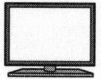 **LEARNING SKILLS, CLEAR PICTURE** WORKSHEET 8

Noticing Thoughts at Different Feelings Levels

Name: _____   Date: _____

Please list thoughts that may go with each feeling and level.

	Rating
Happy	_____
Love	_____
Sad	_____
Confused	_____
Fear	_____
Dislike	_____
Bored	_____
Shame	_____
Anger	_____

_____

_____

_____

_____

_____

_____

_____

_____

_____

From *The Emotion Regulation Skills System Workbook, Second Edition*. Copyright © 2026 Julie F. Brown. Published by The Guilford Press. Permission to photocopy this material or download it from the epdf is granted to purchasers of this book for personal use; see copyright page for details.

| LEARNING SKILLS, CLEAR PICTURE | WORKED EXAMPLE 8 |

Thoughts and Feelings Lead to Urges

Name: _____ Date: _____

Situations can lead us to have thoughts and feelings that lead to action urges.

Thoughts

Situation → Action urge

Feelings and rating

Thoughts
<u>I really liked him.</u>

Situation
<u>Broke up with
my boyfriend.</u>
→ Action urge
<u>Cry.</u>

Feelings and rating
<u>Sadness—Level 3</u>

From *The Emotion Regulation Skills System Workbook, Second Edition.* Copyright © 2026 Julie F. Brown. Published by The Guilford Press. Permission to photocopy this material or download it from the epdf is granted to purchasers of this book for personal use; see copyright page for details.

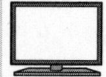 **LEARNING SKILLS, CLEAR PICTURE** **WORKSHEET 9**

Thoughts and Feelings Lead to Urges

Name: _____   Date: _____

Situations can lead us to have thoughts and feelings that lead to action urges.

Thoughts

Situation → Action urge

Feelings and rating

Thoughts
_____

Situation _____ → Action urge _____

Feelings and rating
_____

From *The Emotion Regulation Skills System Workbook, Second Edition*. Copyright © 2026 Julie F. Brown. Published by The Guilford Press. Permission to photocopy this material or download it from the epdf is granted to purchasers of this book for personal use; see copyright page for details.

LEARNING SKILLS, CLEAR PICTURE **WORKED EXAMPLE 9**

Feelings and Their Action Urges

Name: _____   Date: _____

Please list action urges that each feeling gives you.

	Happy	*Clap my hands*
	Love	*Hug*
	Sad	*Look down*
	Confused	*Avoid*
	Fear	*Scream*
	Dislike	*Move away*
	Bored	*Complain*
	Shame	*Hide*
	Anger	*Yell*

From *The Emotion Regulation Skills System Workbook, Second Edition*. Copyright © 2026 Julie F. Brown. Published by The Guilford Press. Permission to photocopy this material or download it from the epdf is granted to purchasers of this book for personal use; see copyright page for details.

LEARNING SKILLS, CLEAR PICTURE WORKSHEET 10

Feelings and Their Action Urges

Name: _____ Date: _____

Please list action urges that each feeling gives you.

Happy _____

Love _____

Sad _____

Confused _____

Fear _____

Dislike _____

Bored _____

Shame _____

Anger _____

From *The Emotion Regulation Skills System Workbook, Second Edition*. Copyright © 2026 Julie F. Brown. Published by The Guilford Press. Permission to photocopy this material or download it from the epdf is granted to purchasers of this book for personal use; see copyright page for details.

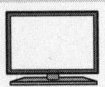 **LEARNING SKILLS, CLEAR PICTURE** — WORKED EXAMPLE 10

Action Urges by Feelings Level

Name: _____ Date: _____

Please choose a feeling and list an action urge for each level.

Emotion: __Anxiety_____

0 — Relaxed

1 — Get fidgety

2 — Talk a lot

3 — Get out of here

4 — Run and find a safe place

5 — Gasp for breath

From *The Emotion Regulation Skills System Workbook, Second Edition*. Copyright © 2026 Julie F. Brown. Published by The Guilford Press. Permission to photocopy this material or download it from the epdf is granted to purchasers of this book for personal use; see copyright page for details.

LEARNING SKILLS, CLEAR PICTURE **WORKSHEET 11**

Action Urges by Feelings Level

Name: _____ Date: _____

Please choose a feeling and list an action urge for each level.

Emotion: _____

0 _____

1 _____

2 _____

3 _____

4 _____

5 _____

From *The Emotion Regulation Skills System Workbook, Second Edition*. Copyright © 2026 Julie F. Brown. Published by The Guilford Press. Permission to photocopy this material or download it from the epdf is granted to purchasers of this book for personal use; see copyright page for details.

LEARNING SKILLS, CLEAR PICTURE WORKED EXAMPLE 11

Situations That Lead to Noticing Urges

Name: _____ Date: _____

Directions: Situations often make us have urges to take action. In Clear Picture we notice our urges before we take action. We don't change urges in Clear Picture—we just notice them. Write down a situation and what you would feel like doing if the situation happened.

Situation: _____Someone said "thank you" to me._____

↘ Urge: _____

Situation: _____Someone didn't say "thank you" to me._____

↘ Urge: _____

Situation: _____It is time for me to exercise._____

↘ Urge: _____

Situation: _____I am at an all-you-can-eat buffet._____

↘ Urge: _____

Situation: _____I got a new phone._____

↘ Urge: _____

From *The Emotion Regulation Skills System Workbook, Second Edition*. Copyright © 2026 Julie F. Brown. Published by The Guilford Press. Permission to photocopy this material or download it from the epdf is granted to purchasers of this book for personal use; see copyright page for details.

LEARNING SKILLS, CLEAR PICTURE　　　　**WORKSHEET 12**

Situations That Lead to Noticing Urges

Name: _____　　Date: _____

Directions: Situations often make us have urges to take action. In Clear Picture we notice our urges before we take action. We don't change urges in Clear Picture—we just notice them. Write down a situation and what you would feel like doing if the situation happened.

Situation: _____
　↘
　　Urge: _____

Situation: _____
　↘
　　Urge: _____

Situation: _____
　↘
　　Urge: _____

Situation: _____
　↘
　　Urge: _____

Situation: _____
　↘
　　Urge: _____

From *The Emotion Regulation Skills System Workbook, Second Edition*. Copyright © 2026 Julie F. Brown. Published by The Guilford Press. Permission to photocopy this material or download it from the epdf is granted to purchasers of this book for personal use; see copyright page for details.

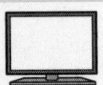 **LEARNING SKILLS, CLEAR PICTURE** **WORKED EXAMPLE 12**

Noticing My Reactions

Name: _____ Date: _____

Directions: Situations make us have thoughts, feelings, and urges to take action. In Clear Picture we notice our urges before we take the action. We don't change urges in Clear Picture—we notice them first. For each of these situations, fill in a thought, feeling, and urge you might have.

Situation: ____Someone ate the rest of my favorite cereal.____

  Thought: ____I really wanted my cereal today.____

    Feeling: ____Disappointed____   Rating: ____2____

      Urge: ____Complain about people I live with.____

Situation: ____I am running 10 minutes late for work.____

  Thought: ____I am going to get in trouble.____

    Feeling: ____Upset____   Rating: ____3____

      Urge: ____Drive really fast.____

Situation: ____A special family member is visiting me today.____

  Thought: ____Missy and I have a lot of fun together.____

    Feeling: ____Excited____   Rating: ____4____

      Urge: ____Pace around until she comes.____

From *The Emotion Regulation Skills System Workbook, Second Edition*. Copyright © 2026 Julie F. Brown. Published by The Guilford Press. Permission to photocopy this material or download it from the epdf is granted to purchasers of this book for personal use; see copyright page for details.

LEARNING SKILLS, CLEAR PICTURE **WORKSHEET 13**

Noticing My Reactions

Name: _____   Date: _____

Directions: Situations make us have thoughts, feelings, and urges to take action. In Clear Picture we notice our urges before we take the action. We don't change urges in Clear Picture—we notice them first. For each of these situations, fill in a thought, feeling, and urge you might have.

Situation: _____

   Thought: _____

     Feeling: _____   Rating: _____

       Urge: _____

Situation: _____

   Thought: _____

     Feeling: _____   Rating: _____

       Urge: _____

Situation: _____

   Thought: _____

     Feeling: _____   Rating: _____

       Urge: _____

From *The Emotion Regulation Skills System Workbook, Second Edition*. Copyright © 2026 Julie F. Brown. Published by The Guilford Press. Permission to photocopy this material or download it from the epdf is granted to purchasers of this book for personal use; see copyright page for details.

On-Track Thinking

LEARNING SKILLS, ON-TRACK THINKING — SUMMARY SHEET

On-Track Thinking

On-Track Thinking is an All-the-Time skill. I use On-Track Thinking at every level of feeling, 0–5.

Once I get a Clear Picture and notice my thoughts and urges in a situation, I begin to do On-Track Thinking. The first step in On-Track Thinking is to **stop** and **Check It**. I *Check it* before I take any action to be sure it will help me reach my goals. I give it a *thumbs up* if it is a helpful thought or urge. Helpful thoughts and urges help me to be on-track to my goals. I give the thought or urge a *thumbs down* if it is off-track. Off-track urges do not help me reach my goals. I try to balance my short-term and long-term needs when I check if something is helpful or not. Thoughts and urges are like city buses; I only get on those that will take me where I want to go.

If the thought or urge is off-track, I **Turn It** to on-track thinking. Instead of having more off-track thoughts, I create on-track thoughts in my mind. I coach myself to head in the right direction. I allow off-track thoughts to pass. If an off-track thought pops back in, I notice it, Turn It, and don't get on that bus!

Once I start on-track thinking, I **Cheerlead.** Off-Track thoughts can come back, so I cheer myself on to stay on-track to my goal even when it is difficult. I tell myself about how I want to stay on-track and not act on urges that would cause negative consequences. I also use Cheerleading to give myself the strength and motivation to get where I want to go. The stronger the off-track thoughts and urges are, the more I need to do Check It, Turn It, and Cheerleading thinking while I make and do my Skills Plan. I get on and stay on the right buses all the way to my goal!

Then I make a Skills Plan.

- My level of feeling 0–1–2–3–4–5 helps me know which skills and how many I need to use.

- I use the Categories of Skills to help me decide which skills I can use. If I am at or below a 3 feeling, I can use all nine skills—even the Calm-Only ones. I have to be focused and thinking clearly when using Problem Solving, Expressing Myself, Getting It Right, and Relationship Care. When I am at or below a 3, I am better able to interact with people in positive ways. I have to be able to talk and listen to use my Calm-Only skills.

If I or the other person are over a 3, even a little bit, I generally use my All-the-Time skills. My All-the-Time skills are Clear Picture, On-Track Thinking, On-Track Action, Safety Plan, and New-Me Activity. I might be ready to interact using Calm-Only skills, but if the other person is over a 3, the situation is likely to go off-track for both of us. I wait until we are both below a 3 to fix problems, express ourselves, use Getting It Right, or do Relationship Care.

- Then I use the Recipe for Skills. The recipe tells me how many skills I need to use. I add one skill to my level of feeling. So, at a 3 feeling, I need to use at least four skills. The higher the feeling level, the more skills I need to chain together, because stronger feelings tend to last longer. The recipe tells me the minimum number of skills to use in a situation. A Skills Master uses more than just the minimum! It is important to remember that if I am at a Level 5 feeling, I can't use my Calm-Only skills. In that situation I have to double-up on All-the-Time skills such as On-Track Actions and New-Me Activities.

- Next, I think about which skills I will use in a situation. I start with Clear Picture and do On-Track Thinking to be sure I take On-Track Actions. If I have a fuzzy picture or off-track thinking, I am likely to take off-track actions. Using Skills 123 together helps me be in Wise Mind. The 123 Wise Mind is for when I am thinking *and* feeling *and* moving toward my goals.

Building Strong Skills Chains

- Wise Mind skills chains start with Skills 1 (Clear Picture), 2 (On-Track Thinking), and 3 (On-Track Action) as the first three links. I add other skills as needed. For example, I add Safety Plan if there is risk. That chain would be a 1234. I add New-Me Activities to help me focus, feel good, distract myself, and have fun. That chain would be a 1235 if I did one New-Me Activity and a 12355 if I did two New-Me Activities. If I do a Safety Plan and two New-Me Activities, it would be a 123455 skills chain. If I am at or below a 3, I may add Problem Solving, Expressing Myself, Getting It Right, and/or Relationship Care as needed to best reach my goals. A Problem Solving skills chain would be a 1236.

From *The Emotion Regulation Skills System Workbook, Second Edition.* Copyright © 2026 Julie F. Brown. Published by The Guilford Press. Permission to photocopy this material or download it from the epdf is granted to purchasers of this book for personal use; see copyright page for details.

LEARNING SKILLS, ON-TRACK THINKING HANDOUT 1

On-Track Thinking to Meet My Goals

Once I have a Clear Picture, I do On-Track Thinking to help me reach my goals.

 **Check It**

Does the urge help me reach my goal?

Helpful 👍   or   👎 Not Helpful?

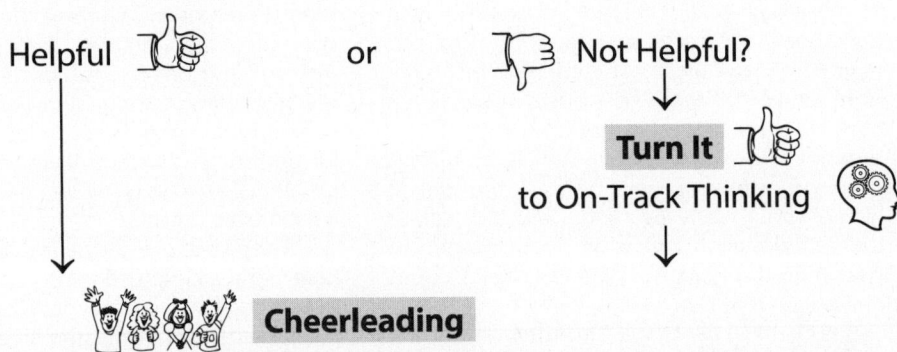

Turn It 👍 to On-Track Thinking

Cheerleading

Cheerleading thoughts coach me to do what works to get me to my goal.

"I don't want to go off-track."
"I want to reach my goal."
"I will make the best of it."
"I can handle this."

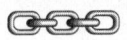 **Make a Skills Plan**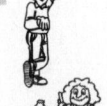

- Can I use Calm-Only skills?

- How many skills do I need?

- What skills will I link together to help me reach my goal?

Take an On-Track Action

From *The Emotion Regulation Skills System Workbook, Second Edition*. Copyright © 2026 Julie F. Brown. Published by The Guilford Press. Permission to photocopy this material or download it from the epdf is granted to purchasers of this book for personal use; see copyright page for details.

| LEARNING SKILLS, ON-TRACK THINKING | WORKED EXAMPLE 1 |

On-Track Thinking Through a Situation

Name: _____ Date: _____

Directions: Think of a situation and practice the parts of On-Track Thinking.

Situation: <u>I am at work and I feel sick.</u>

✓ Check It

I have the urge to <u>quit my job.</u>

Is the urge HELPFUL? 👍 or (👎) NOT HELPFUL to reach my goal?

👍 Turn It to On-Track Thinking

<u>I need this job!</u>

🎉 Cheerleading

<u>I quit my last job and that didn't work out well.</u>
<u>I can deal with this even though I am miserable.</u>

🔗 Make a Skills Plan

I am at a: 0–1–2–③–4–5

Can I use Calm-Only skills now? (YES) or NO

How many skills do I need to use (at least)? <u>4</u>

What skills will I link together to help me reach my goal?

My plan: <u>I will use Clear Picture to know what is going on inside and out.</u>
<u>I will use On-Track Thinking to make a skills plan.</u>
<u>I will use Getting It Right to see if I can go home early.</u>

🚂 On-Track Action

<u>I will go talk to my boss.</u>

From *The Emotion Regulation Skills System Workbook, Second Edition.* Copyright © 2026 Julie F. Brown. Published by The Guilford Press. Permission to photocopy this material or download it from the epdf is granted to purchasers of this book for personal use; see copyright page for details.

LEARNING SKILLS, ON-TRACK THINKING

WORKSHEET 1

On-Track Thinking Through a Situation

Name: _____ Date: _____

Directions: Think of a situation and practice the parts of On-Track Thinking.

Situation: _____

✓ Check It

I have the urge to _____

Is the urge HELPFUL? 👍 or 👎 NOT HELPFUL to reach my goal?

👍 Turn It to On-Track Thinking

_____

Cheerleading

_____

_____

_____

Make a Skills Plan

I am at a: 0–1–2–3–4–5

Can I use Calm-Only skills now?   YES or NO

How many skills do I need to use (at least)? _____

What skills will I link together to help me reach my goal?

My plan: _____

_____

On-Track Action

From *The Emotion Regulation Skills System Workbook, Second Edition*. Copyright © 2026 Julie F. Brown. Published by The Guilford Press. Permission to photocopy this material or download it from the epdf is granted to purchasers of this book for personal use; see copyright page for details.

LEARNING SKILLS, ON-TRACK THINKING | **WORKSHEET 2**

Check It

Name: _____ Date: _____

Does the urge help me reach my goal?

👍 = 🚂 On-Track Urges

👎 = 💥🚂 Off-Track Urges

Please think about your personal goals.

Circle whether the urge is helpful 👍 or not helpful. 👎

1. I feel like hitting that girl. 👍 👎

2. I want to focus in group. 👍 👎

3. I want to drive too fast. 👍 👎

4. I want to steal a phone. 👍 👎

5. I want to be healthy. 👍 👎

6. I want to put myself down. 👍 👎

7. I want to make some new friends. 👍 👎

8. I want to scream at my teacher. 👍 👎

From *The Emotion Regulation Skills System Workbook, Second Edition*. Copyright © 2026 Julie F. Brown. Published by The Guilford Press. Permission to photocopy this material or download it from the epdf is granted to purchasers of this book for personal use; see copyright page for details.

| LEARNING SKILLS, ON-TRACK THINKING | WORKED EXAMPLE 2 |

Turn It

Name: _____ Date: _____

From Off-Track to On-Track Thinking

Directions: Think of a goal. Then think of urges that either help you or don't help you reach the goal. Write down the urge, Check It, Turn It, and write four Cheerleading statements that will support you to reach this goal.

To Check It and Turn It, I have to take a second to think about my goal in the situation.

Goal: *I want my own apartment.*

Urge: *I don't want to do my laundry.*

Check It 👍 or 👎

Turn It *I need to do my laundry.*

Cheerleading
If I wear dirty clothes I will look terrible.
I want to be a clean person and look good.
I want to be independent and responsible.
I will feel better when it is done.

From *The Emotion Regulation Skills System Workbook, Second Edition.* Copyright © 2026 Julie F. Brown. Published by The Guilford Press. Permission to photocopy this material or download it from the epdf is granted to purchasers of this book for personal use; see copyright page for details.

LEARNING SKILLS, ON-TRACK THINKING **WORKSHEET 3**

Turn It

Name: _____ Date: _____

From Off-Track to On-Track Thinking

Directions: Think of a goal. Then think of urges that either help you or don't help you reach the goal. Write down the urge, Check It, Turn It, and write four Cheerleading statements that will support you to reach this goal.

To Check It and Turn It, I have to take a second to think about my goal in the situation.

Goal: _____

Urge: _____ Check It

👍 or 👎

👍 Turn It _____

🙌 Cheerleading _____

_____

_____

_____

From *The Emotion Regulation Skills System Workbook, Second Edition*. Copyright © 2026 Julie F. Brown. Published by The Guilford Press. Permission to photocopy this material or download it from the epdf is granted to purchasers of this book for personal use; see copyright page for details.

LEARNING SKILLS, ON-TRACK THINKING **WORKED EXAMPLE 3**

On-Track Thinking: Create a Skills Plan

Name: _____ Date: _____

Directions: Please create your own Skills Plan.

Situation: <u>I am upset at Missy because she canceled our visit.</u>
_____

My breath: <u>Shallow and fast.</u>
My body check: <u>My fists are tight and I have a stomachache.</u>
My surroundings: <u>I am in my bedroom.</u>
_____

My feeling: <u>Hurt</u>   Rating level: <u>4</u>.
My thought: <u>She always cancels our visits.</u>
My urge: <u>Call Missy and yell at her.</u>

Next, I Checked it. My thoughts/urges were ____ ON-TRACK or <u>X</u> OFF-TRACK.

   If off-track, my Turn It thought was: <u>I want to be Missy's friend.</u>
   <u>Yelling at her will harm our friendship.</u>

My Cheerleading statements: <u>She is sick so it makes sense she canceled</u>
<u>the visit. I want to be understanding and support her.</u>

I made a Skills Plan. Because I was at a level <u>4</u> of feeling, I could use my

   (**All-the-Time Skills**)   **Calm-Only Skills**

How many skills did I have to use *at least*? <u>5</u>

What skills could I link together in this situation?

From *The Emotion Regulation Skills System Workbook, Second Edition*. Copyright © 2026 Julie F. Brown. Published by The Guilford Press. Permission to photocopy this material or download it from the epdf is granted to purchasers of this book for personal use; see copyright page for details.

| LEARNING SKILLS, ON-TRACK THINKING | WORKSHEET 4 |

On-Track Thinking: Create a Skills Plan

Name: _____   Date: _____

Directions: Please create your own Skills Plan.

Situation: _____
_____

My breath: _____
My body check: _____
My surroundings: _____
_____

My feeling: _____ Rating level: _____.
My thought: _____
My urge: _____

Next, I Checked it. My thoughts/urges were _____ ON-TRACK or _____ OFF-TRACK.

    If off-track, my Turn It thought was: _____
_____

My Cheerleading statements: _____
_____

I made a Skills Plan. Because I was at a level _____ of feeling, I could use my

        All-the-Time Skills   **Calm-Only Skills**

How many skills did I have to use *at least*? _____

What skills could I link together in this situation?

From *The Emotion Regulation Skills System Workbook, Second Edition*. Copyright © 2026 Julie F. Brown. Published by The Guilford Press. Permission to photocopy this material or download it from the epdf is granted to purchasers of this book for personal use; see copyright page for details.

| LEARNING SKILLS, ON-TRACK THINKING | WORKED EXAMPLE 4 |

Cheerleading: Blast It

Name: _____ Date: _____

Directions: At times off-track thoughts and urges can increase our uncomfortable emotions and raise our feelings ratings to 4–5's when that is not our goal. Cheerleading statements are often sprinkled throughout our skills chains to encourage us and to keep us on-track. Sometimes sprinkling isn't enough—we need a strong and continuous blast of on-track thoughts and cheers that help us reframe persistent off-track thoughts and urges.

Write down a situation that often causes you to struggle. List at least 10 Cheerleading statements that encourage you. Perhaps remind yourself of things like:

- Feelings come and go—they don't last forever!
- By using skills, I can feel better!
- I can manage the situation!
- I have handled challenges before, and I was OK!
- I have resources that can help me, like New-Me Activities, relationships, and my spirituality.

Read your Blast It list over and over when you need a blast of On-Track Thinking. Make new Blast It lists as you think of new ways to encourage yourself and to Blast Cheerleading in other situations.

Situation _____ I miss my family. _____

Cheerleading Statements

Maybe I will see or talk to them soon.

I miss them because I love them—That's a good thing.

I can miss them and still be OK.

Sometimes we have to wait for things.

I can wait and be miserable or I can wait and be happy.

I can do things to feel a little better.

This won't last forever. It will pass.

I am not alone.

My family is in my heart.

I have friends who I can call and hang out with.

From *The Emotion Regulation Skills System Workbook, Second Edition*. Copyright © 2026 Julie F. Brown. Published by The Guilford Press. Permission to photocopy this material or download it from the epdf is granted to purchasers of this book for personal use; see copyright page for details.

LEARNING SKILLS, ON-TRACK THINKING — WORKSHEET 5

Cheerleading: Blast It

Name: _____ Date: _____

Directions: At times off-track thoughts and urges can increase our uncomfortable emotions and raise our feelings ratings to 4–5's when that is not our goal. Cheerleading statements are often sprinkled throughout our skills chains to encourage us and to keep us on-track. Sometimes sprinkling isn't enough—we need a strong and continuous blast of on-track thoughts and cheers that help us reframe persistent off-track thoughts and urges.

Write down a situation that often causes you to struggle. List at least 10 Cheerleading statements that encourage you. Perhaps remind yourself of things like:

• Feelings come and go—they don't last forever!
• By using skills, I can feel better!
• I can manage the situation!
• I have handled challenges before, and I was OK!
• I have resources that can help me, like New-Me Activities, relationships, and my spirituality.

Read your Blast It list over and over when you need a blast of On-Track Thinking. Make new Blast It lists as you think of new ways to encourage yourself and to Blast Cheerleading in other situations.

Situation _____

Cheerleading Statements

_____
_____
_____
_____
_____
_____
_____
_____
_____
_____
_____

From *The Emotion Regulation Skills System Workbook, Second Edition*. Copyright © 2026 Julie F. Brown. Published by The Guilford Press. Permission to photocopy this material or download it from the epdf is granted to purchasers of this book for personal use; see copyright page for details.

LEARNING SKILLS, ON-TRACK THINKING **WORKED EXAMPLE 5**

Using Skills in My Life

Name: _____   Date: _____

Directions: List situations or places where it would be helpful to use each skill.

Skill	Situations
Clear Picture	I come home from work
	I wake up in the morning
On-Track Thinking	I want to yell at Jim
	At work
On-Track Action	I'm tired in the morning
	I'm on the phone with family
Safety Plan	Frustrated at work
	People get too close to me
New-Me Activities	Go out on the weekend
	Play solitaire when I'm upset
Problem Solving	Get a new place to live
	See my family more
Expressing Myself	Show my family I care for them
	Share with my friends
Getting It Right	More hours at work
	A date with Sam
Relationship Care	Take good care of myself
	Send cards at the holidays

From *The Emotion Regulation Skills System Workbook, Second Edition*. Copyright © 2026 Julie F. Brown. Published by The Guilford Press. Permission to photocopy this material or download it from the epdf is granted to purchasers of this book for personal use; see copyright page for details.

LEARNING SKILLS, ON-TRACK THINKING WORKSHEET 6

Using Skills in My Life

Name: _____ Date: _____

Directions: List situations or places where it would be helpful to use each skill.

Skill	Situations
Clear Picture	_____
On-Track Thinking	_____
On-Track Action	_____
Safety Plan	_____
New-Me Activities	_____
Problem Solving	_____
Expressing Myself	_____
Getting It Right	_____
Relationship Care	_____

From *The Emotion Regulation Skills System Workbook, Second Edition*. Copyright © 2026 Julie F. Brown. Published by The Guilford Press. Permission to photocopy this material or download it from the epdf is granted to purchasers of this book for personal use; see copyright page for details.

LEARNING SKILLS, ON-TRACK THINKING **WORKED EXAMPLE 6**

Pros and Cons of Using Skills

Name: _____ Date: _____

Directions: When we have a feeling, we think about "Should I do something about this feeling or not?" This worksheet helps us make choices whether to use skills or not to use skills in situations. Write in two situations and list the pros (positive outcomes for you) and cons (negative outcomes for you) of using skills in each one.

Situation _____ I am frustrated with a coworker. _____

Pros of Using Skills
_____ I will keep my job. _____
_____ I will still have a good day. _____

Cons of Using Skills
_____ I won't be able to yell at them and storm out. _____
_____ I will have to focus on my job when I feel like venting. _____

Situation _____ I am lonely. _____

Pros of Using Skills
_____ I can do things to feel less lonely. _____
_____ I can change my life to be around people more. _____

Cons of Using Skills
_____ I am nervous about reaching out to people. _____
_____ I may have to try new things. _____

LEARNING SKILLS, ON-TRACK THINKING **WORKSHEET 7**

Pros and Cons of Using Skills

Name: _____ Date: _____

Directions: When we have a feeling, we think about "Should I do something about this feeling or not?" This worksheet helps us make choices whether to use skills or not to use skills in situations. Write in two situations and list the pros (positive outcomes for you) and cons (negative outcomes for you) of using skills in each one.

Situation _____

Pros of Using Skills

_____

_____

Cons of Using Skills

_____

_____

Situation _____

Pros of Using Skills

_____

_____

Cons of Using Skills

_____

_____

From *The Emotion Regulation Skills System Workbook, Second Edition*. Copyright © 2026 Julie F. Brown. Published by The Guilford Press. Permission to photocopy this material or download it from the epdf is granted to purchasers of this book for personal use; see copyright page for details.

On-Track Action

LEARNING SKILLS, ON-TRACK ACTION — SUMMARY SHEET

On-Track Action

On-Track Action is an All-the-Time skill. This means that I can use On-Track Action at any level of feeling, 0–1–2–3–4–5. First, I get a Clear Picture, then I do On-Track Thinking. I Check It, Turn It, Cheerlead, and make a Skills Plan. Once I have made an On-Track Skills Plan, I decide what my On-Track Action will be. When I do Skills 123, it helps me be in Wise Mind.

I use On-Track Action when I **Take a Step toward My Goal.** I do something to be on-track. For example, if it is my goal to not get into an argument, I may move to my room as part of a Safety Plan or turn on my radio when I want to do a New-Me Activity. I choose to do an On-Track Action to stay on-track to my goals.

I **Switch Tracks** when I need to use a different skill. For example, if I go over a 3 using a Getting It Right, I will have to Switch Tracks to use an All-the-Time skill instead. I also use Switch Tracks when I have urges to go off-track but do something on-track instead. We all go off-track, and it is important to get back on-track as soon as possible—ASAP! The longer I wait, the more difficult it may be. I realize when I am off-track and do several On-Track Actions to be on the right road to my goals.

I may choose to give 100% effort to an On-Track Action. I **Jump in with Both Feet** to an On-Track Action rather than going halfway. When one foot is on-track and the other is off-track, I am still off-track. Sometimes I do the opposite of off-track urges to make sure I am really on-track. For example, I do **Opposite Action** if I feel like avoiding work; instead, I give work 100% effort. Even though it might be hard, I give 100% effort and focus to the On-Track Action.

I make and follow **On-Track Action Plans** to help myself stay on-track. I do things to keep myself and my life in balance. When my body is in balance, I am able to manage life and relationships better. I balance my eating, exercise, health, work, and have fun. For example: I may take walks, get enough sleep, eat healthy food, take proper medications, go to work, and talk to friends as part of my On-Track Action Plan each day.

There are times when I do On-Track Action— **Accept the Situation.** When I have done all I can and I have to wait for the situation to change, I may have to Accept the Situation. For example, if I start fixing a problem and my feelings level goes up, I may have to step back and do On-Track Action— Accept the Situation. I may have to accept when I am over a 3 feeling and need to wait before using Calm-Only skills. It may be important to fix the problem, but waiting until a time when I can do it in an on-track way is best. Also, there are times when I have to do things I don't want to do. I may have to Accept the Situation and jump in with both feet to get it done. Plus, sometimes it isn't possible to change difficult situations. People may say things to me or things may happen to me that I don't like. I have to do what I can to make it better and then maybe do On-Track Action—Accept the Situation. Life gives us plenty of lemons, I have to make lots of lemonade.

There are times when I have to **Turn the Page,** let it go, and move on. I may have the urge to hang on to certain thoughts, feelings, memories, and urges to the point where it begins to cause me a problem. I have to pay attention to when I think "enough is enough" in this situation. I have to be careful to focus on things that help me and to notice when it is no longer helpful. At that point, I may need to do On-Track Action—Turn the Page and move on toward my goals.

From *The Emotion Regulation Skills System Workbook, Second Edition.* Copyright © 2026 Julie F. Brown. Published by The Guilford Press. Permission to photocopy this material or download it from the epdf is granted to purchasers of this book for personal use; see copyright page for details.

LEARNING SKILLS, ON-TRACK ACTION HANDOUT 1

On- and Off-Tracks

I use skills to stay on-track and to get back on-track when I go off-track.

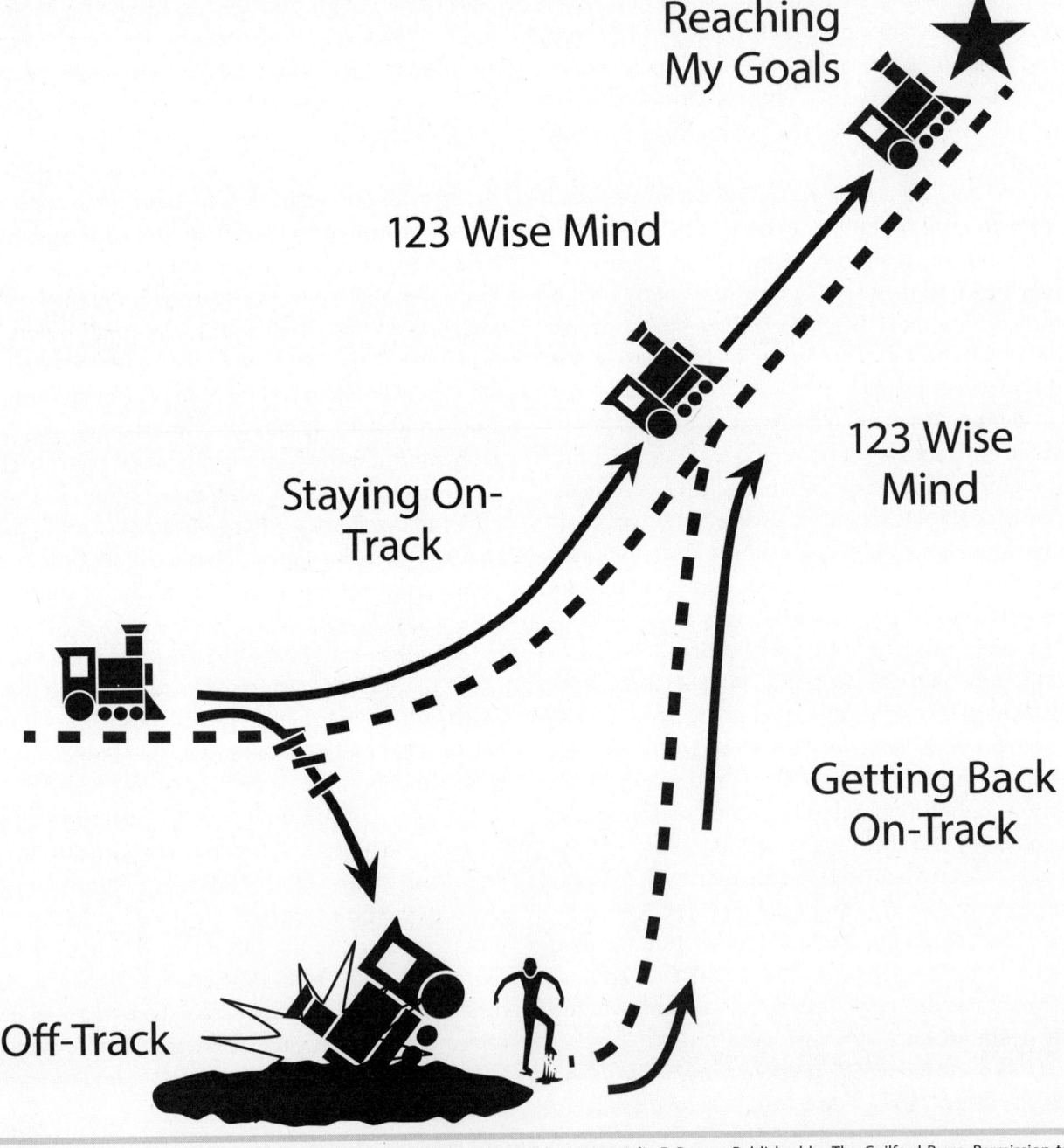

From *The Emotion Regulation Skills System Workbook, Second Edition.* Copyright © 2026 Julie F. Brown. Published by The Guilford Press. Permission to photocopy this material or download it from the epdf is granted to purchasers of this book for personal use; see copyright page for details.

LEARNING SKILLS, ON-TRACK ACTION HANDOUT 2

Five Types of On-Track Actions

These are five different types of On-Track Actions. We may use more than one type of On-Track Action in a situation. For example, we may Switch Tracks AND Take a Step toward Our Goals. We may even use all five in a situation. We do what works!

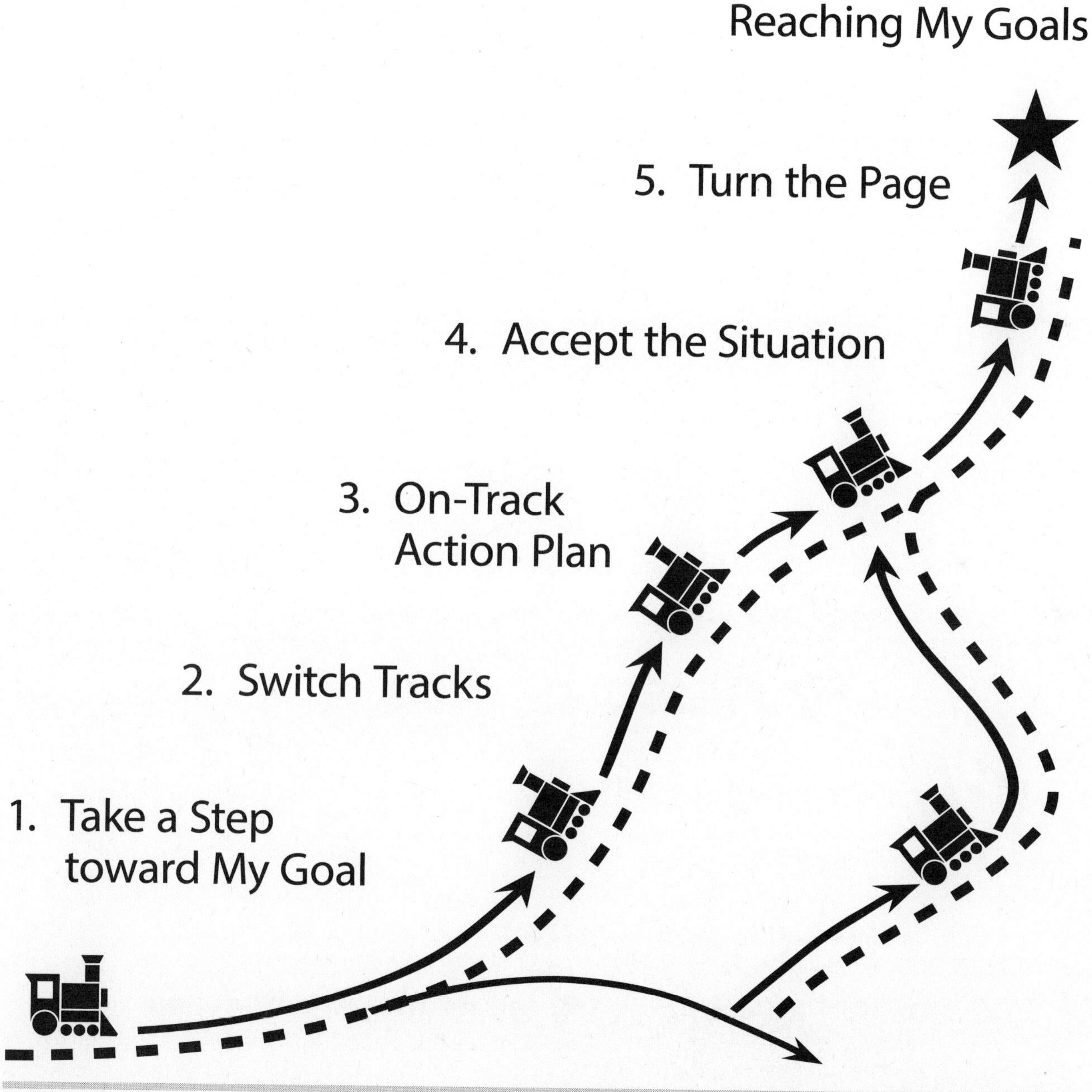

Reaching My Goals

5. Turn the Page

4. Accept the Situation

3. On-Track Action Plan

2. Switch Tracks

1. Take a Step toward My Goal

From *The Emotion Regulation Skills System Workbook, Second Edition.* Copyright © 2026 Julie F. Brown. Published by The Guilford Press. Permission to photocopy this material or download it from the epdf is granted to purchasers of this book for personal use; see copyright page for details.

LEARNING SKILLS, ON-TRACK ACTION

HANDOUT 3

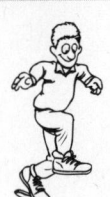

Take a Step toward My Goal in Wise Mind

0–1–2–3–4–5
I can step to:
3. On-Track Action
4. Safety Plan
5. New-Me Activity

0–1–2–3
I can also step to:
6. Problem Solving
7. Expressing Myself
8. Getting It Right
9. Relationship Care

Goal: "I want to be safe"

5. New-Me Activity: Play solitaire

4. Safety Plan—Move away

3. On-Track Action

2. On-Track Thinking

1. Clear Picture

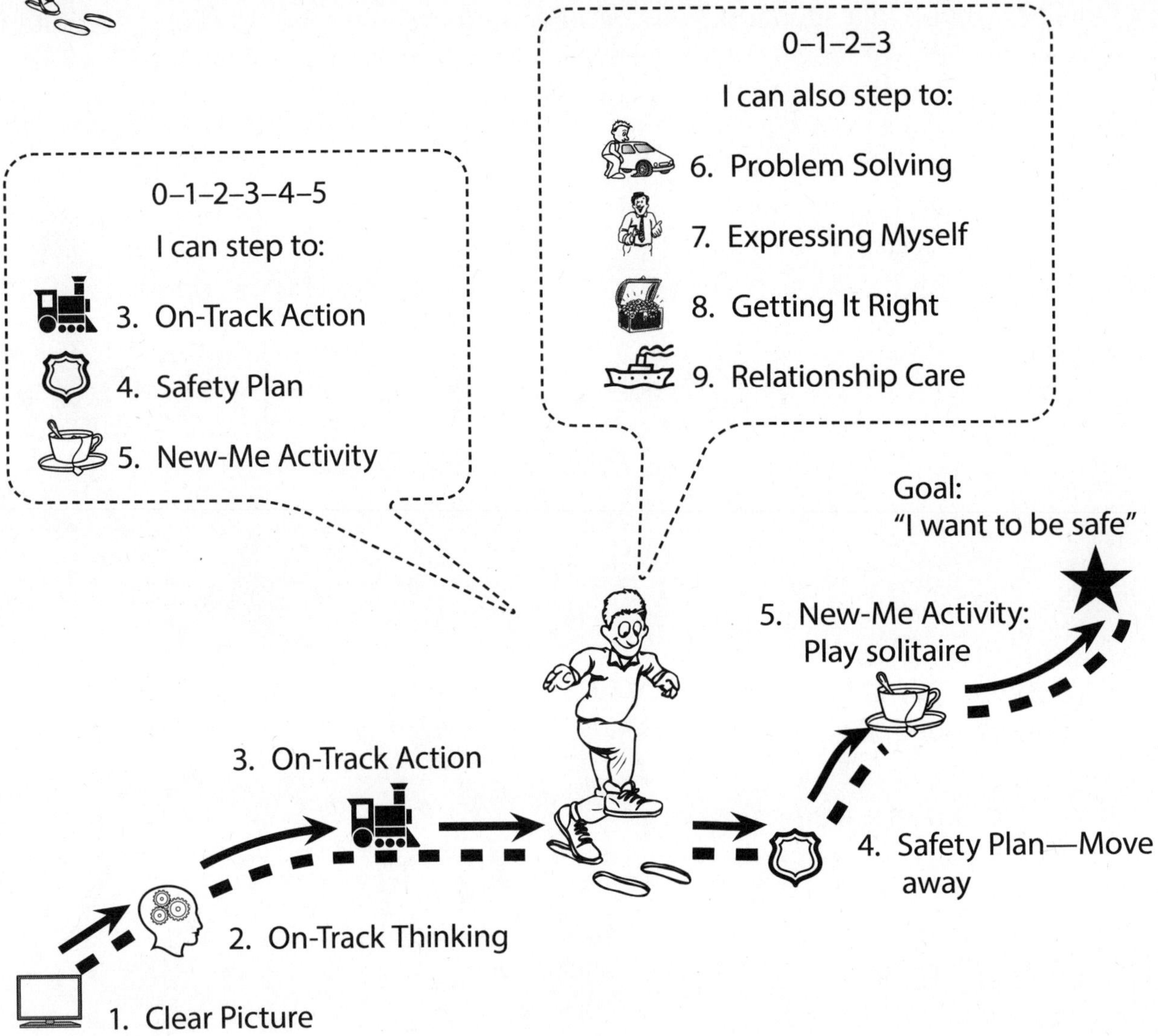

On-Track Action—Take a Step toward My Goal in Wise Mind

From *The Emotion Regulation Skills System Workbook, Second Edition*. Copyright © 2026 Julie F. Brown. Published by The Guilford Press. Permission to photocopy this material or download it from the epdf is granted to purchasers of this book for personal use; see copyright page for details.

LEARNING SKILLS, ON-TRACK ACTION **WORKED EXAMPLE 1**

On-Track Actions and My Goals

Name: _____ Date: _____

Directions: Under the On-Track Actions heading, list actions that will likely help you reach My Goals. In the right column, write down My Goals that the On-Track Actions will help you reach.

On-Track Actions	**My Goals**
Encourage myself →	Use my skills
Take a walk in nature →	Be healthy
Go to work →	Have money to buy things
Take my medications →	Be healthy
Hang out with friends →	Be happy
Do my chores →	Be independent
Go to bed by 10 pm →	Be healthy
Visit my family →	Be happy

From *The Emotion Regulation Skills System Workbook, Second Edition.* Copyright © 2026 Julie F. Brown. Published by The Guilford Press. Permission to photocopy this material or download it from the epdf is granted to purchasers of this book for personal use; see copyright page for details.

LEARNING SKILLS, ON-TRACK ACTION **WORKSHEET 1**

On-Track Actions and My Goals

Name: _____   Date: _____

Directions: Under the On-Track Actions heading, list actions that will likely help you reach My Goals. In the right column, write down My Goals that the On-Track Actions will help you reach.

On-Track Actions	**My Goals**
———————————→	———————————
———————————→	———————————
———————————→	———————————
———————————→	———————————
———————————→	———————————
———————————→	———————————
———————————→	———————————

From *The Emotion Regulation Skills System Workbook, Second Edition*. Copyright © 2026 Julie F. Brown. Published by The Guilford Press. Permission to photocopy this material or download it from the epdf is granted to purchasers of this book for personal use; see copyright page for details.

LEARNING SKILLS, ON-TRACK ACTION **HANDOUT 4**

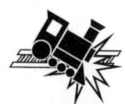 # Switch Tracks to On-Track Action

"I'm really tired. It is cold. I don't like the cold. I don't want to get up."

"Not helpful! I need to get up and go to work!"

"A shower is a New-Me Activity right now! I will jump in."

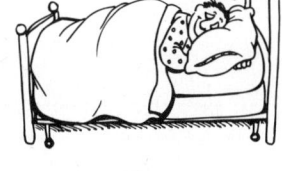 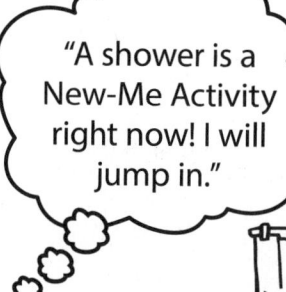

1. Clear Picture
2. On-Track Thinking
3. **On-Track Action!**

Helpful Hints:

Jump On-Track with Both Feet!

I give 100% effort and focus to my On-Track Action.

One foot off-track and one on-track is still off-track!

Do the Opposite Action of Off-Track Urges!

Doing an Opposite Action can help me get used to things I want to avoid. If I would like to dance but avoid it because I am afraid, I do the opposite. I take lessons and ask people to dance. Opposite Action can make me feel good things I tend to avoid.

From *The Emotion Regulation Skills System Workbook, Second Edition*. Copyright © 2026 Julie F. Brown. Published by The Guilford Press. Permission to photocopy this material or download it from the epdf is granted to purchasers of this book for personal use; see copyright page for details.

LEARNING SKILLS, ON-TRACK ACTION **WORKED EXAMPLE 2**

On-Track Action: Switching Tracks

Name: _____   Date: _____

Directions: Under the Off-Track Actions heading, list actions that will likely take you off-track. In the right column, write down an On-Track Action that would help you Switch Tracks. Doing the Opposite of Off-Track Actions can help us get back on-track and help us stay on-track in the future.

Off-Track Actions	On-Track Actions to My New-Me
Put myself down	Treat myself with kindness
Worry a lot	Trust things will work out OK
Punch a wall	Take a walk
Skip my medications	Take medications on time
Cheat at a game	Play to have fun—win or lose
Tell my teacher off	Set up a meeting to talk
Drink too much soda	Get a water bottle
Watch too much TV	Go out with friends

From *The Emotion Regulation Skills System Workbook, Second Edition*. Copyright © 2026 Julie F. Brown. Published by The Guilford Press. Permission to photocopy this material or download it from the epdf is granted to purchasers of this book for personal use; see copyright page for details.

LEARNING SKILLS, ON-TRACK ACTION **WORKSHEET 2**

On-Track Action: Switching Tracks

Name: _____   Date: _____

Directions: Under the Off-Track Actions heading, list actions that will likely take you off-track. In the right column, write down an On-Track Action that would help you Switch Tracks. Doing the Opposite of Off-Track Actions can help us get back on-track and help us stay on-track in the future.

Off-Track Actions	**On-Track Actions to My New-Me**
──────────────→	──────────────
──────────────→	──────────────
──────────────→	──────────────
──────────────→	──────────────
──────────────→	──────────────
──────────────→	──────────────
──────────────→	──────────────

From *The Emotion Regulation Skills System Workbook, Second Edition*. Copyright © 2026 Julie F. Brown. Published by The Guilford Press. Permission to photocopy this material or download it from the epdf is granted to purchasers of this book for personal use; see copyright page for details.

LEARNING SKILLS, ON-TRACK ACTION HANDOUT 5

On-Track Action Plans

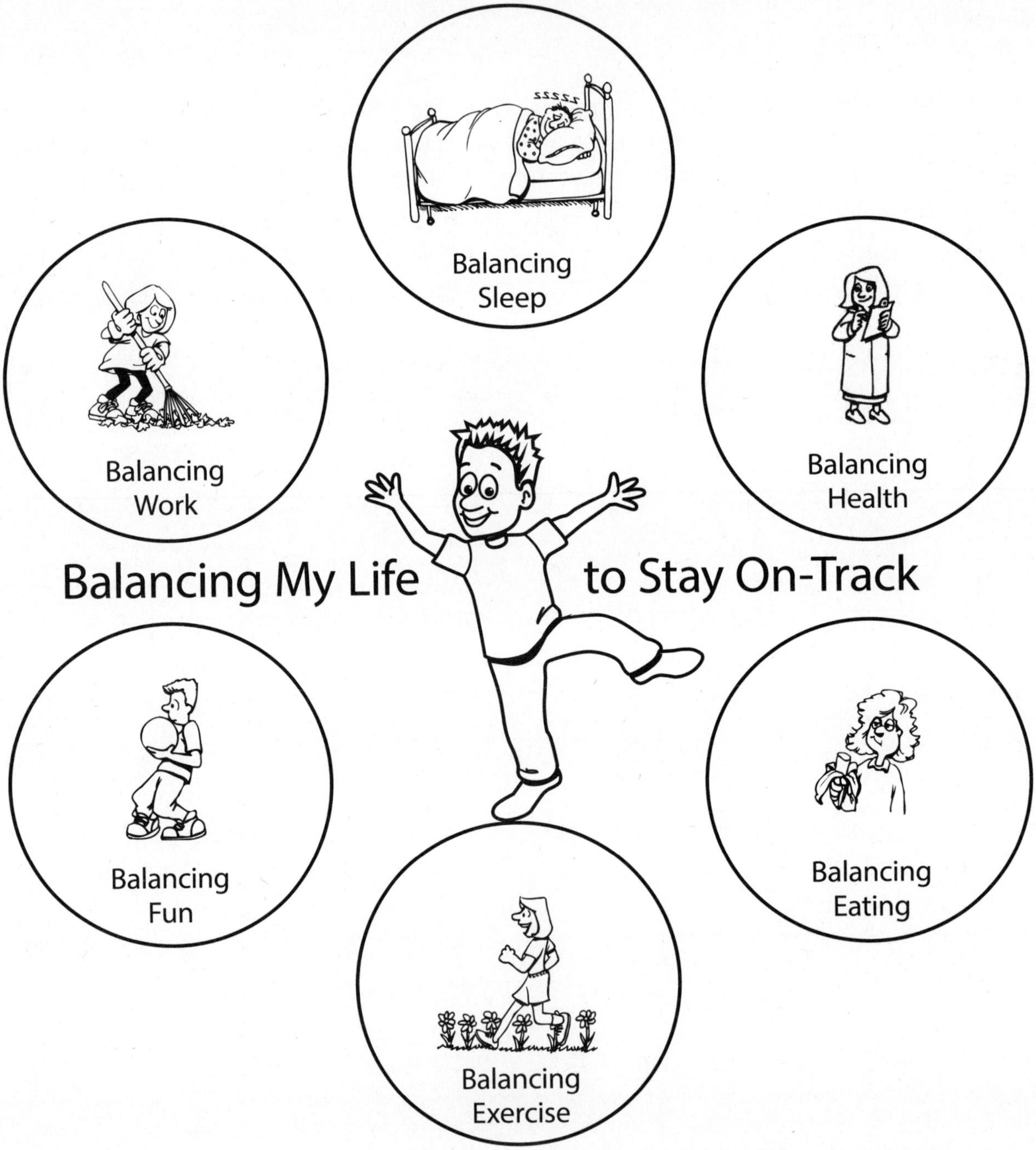

- Balancing Sleep
- Balancing Work
- Balancing Health
- Balancing Fun
- Balancing Eating
- Balancing Exercise

Balancing My Life to Stay On-Track

From *The Emotion Regulation Skills System Workbook, Second Edition.* Copyright © 2026 Julie F. Brown. Published by The Guilford Press. Permission to photocopy this material or download it from the epdf is granted to purchasers of this book for personal use; see copyright page for details.

LEARNING SKILLS, ON-TRACK ACTION **WORKED EXAMPLE 3**

My On-Track Action Plan

Name: _____   Date: _____

Please list what you do to balance your life and stay on-track.

Balancing Eating: I eat three healthy meals a day. I eat fruit for snacks. I don't eat junk food very much. I try to have low-fat things and salads.

Balancing Exercise: I try to take a walk every day. I go on the treadmill when there is bad weather. I stretch my muscles and do a few yoga poses.

Balancing Sleep: I try to go to bed by 10:00 at night. I get up at 6:00 in the morning. That is 8 hours of sleep per night. I take naps if I am very tired.

Balancing Health: I get a checkup every year. I go to the doctor when I need to. I talk with my doctor about my concerns. I take my medications.

Balancing Work: I do many chores in my house. I put in three job applications per week. I do volunteer work to keep busy and to get work experience.

Balancing Fun: I try to do something fun every day. I like to take walks, talk to friends, cook food, watch TV, listen to the radio, and help out around the house.

From *The Emotion Regulation Skills System Workbook, Second Edition.* Copyright © 2026 Julie F. Brown. Published by The Guilford Press. Permission to photocopy this material or download it from the epdf is granted to purchasers of this book for personal use; see copyright page for details.

| LEARNING SKILLS, ON-TRACK ACTION | WORKSHEET 3 |

My On-Track Action Plan

Name: _____   Date: _____

Please list what you do to balance your life and stay on-track.

Balancing Eating: _____
_____
_____

Balancing Exercise: _____
_____
_____

Balancing Sleep: _____
_____
_____

Balancing Health: _____
_____
_____

Balancing Work: _____
_____
_____

Balancing Fun: _____
_____
_____

From *The Emotion Regulation Skills System Workbook, Second Edition*. Copyright © 2026 Julie F. Brown. Published by The Guilford Press. Permission to photocopy this material or download it from the epdf is granted to purchasers of this book for personal use; see copyright page for details.

LEARNING SKILLS, ON-TRACK ACTION   **WORKSHEET 4**

Balancing in My Life

Name: _____   Date: _____

Directions: In the circles below, list aspects of your life that you strive to balance. Some examples are: "family," "self-care," "spirituality," "screen-time," "emailing," "social media," "relationships," "chores," "work," "fitness," "TV," "eating," "drinking," "sleeping," "socializing," and/or "spending money."

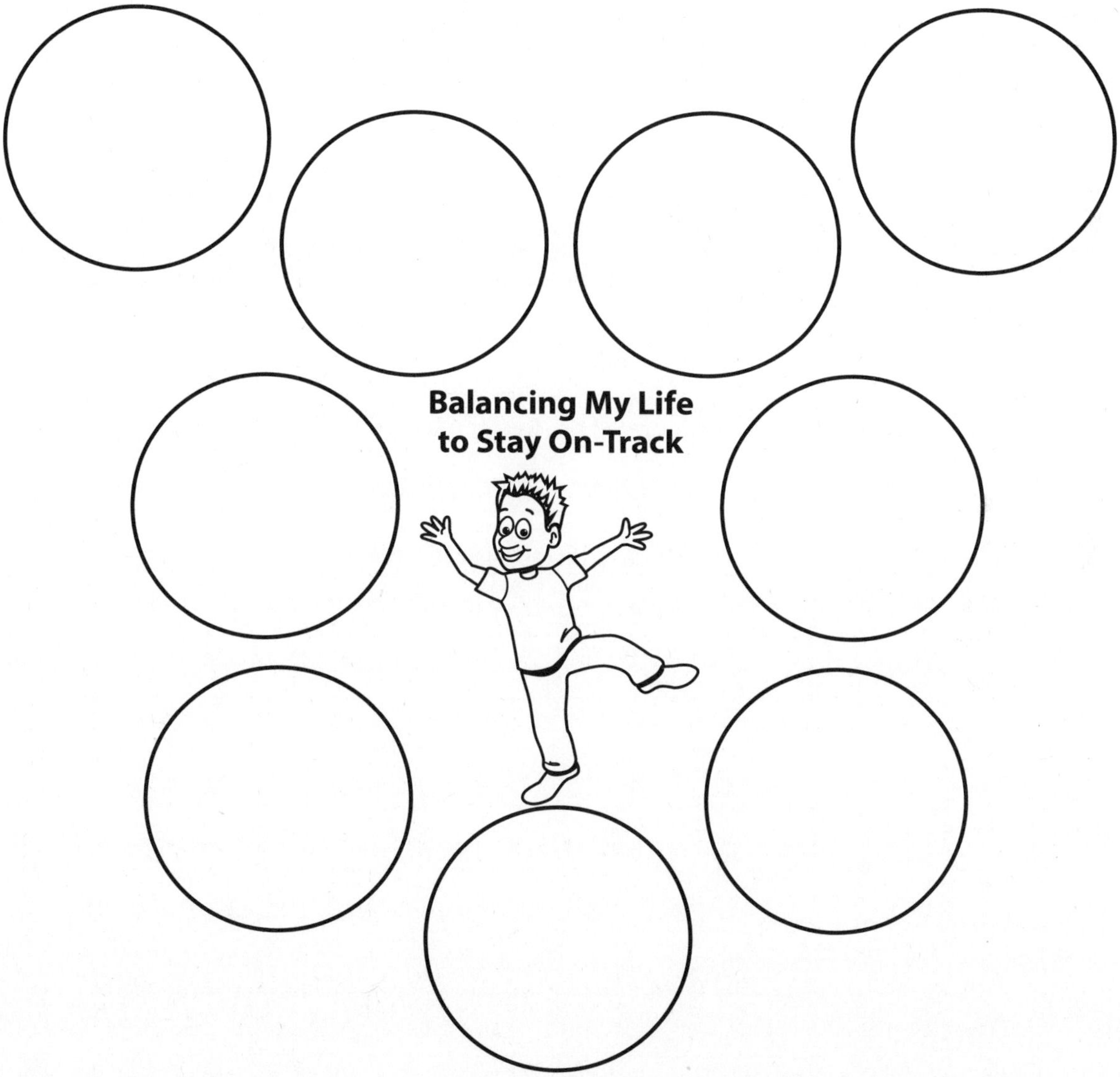

Balancing My Life to Stay On-Track

From *The Emotion Regulation Skills System Workbook, Second Edition*. Copyright © 2026 Julie F. Brown. Published by The Guilford Press. Permission to photocopy this material or download it from the epdf is granted to purchasers of this book for personal use; see copyright page for details.

LEARNING SKILLS, ON-TRACK ACTION — WORKED EXAMPLE 4

Balancing My Life

Name: _____   Date: _____

Directions: Write one, two, or three aspects of your life you would like to balance from My On-Track Action Plan (Worksheet 3) in the circles below. List several On-Track Actions that will help you actively balance each aspect.

Aspects to Balance   **On-Track Actions**

(Pass my class.)
- Go to class.
- Stay awake and take notes.
- Ask questions in class.
- Study for tests.

(Get enough exercise.)
- Exercise 5 days per week.
- Block out time for walks.
- Listen to music when I exercise.
- Ask a friend to walk with me.

(Get enough sleep.)
- Go to bed at 10 pm and get up at 7 am.
- Don't watch upsetting TV shows before bed.
- Don't be on my phone after 8 pm.
- Don't nap too much during the day.

From *The Emotion Regulation Skills System Workbook, Second Edition*. Copyright © 2026 Julie F. Brown. Published by The Guilford Press. Permission to photocopy this material or download it from the epdf is granted to purchasers of this book for personal use; see copyright page for details.

| LEARNING SKILLS, ON-TRACK ACTION | **WORKSHEET 5** |

Balancing My Life

Name: _____ Date: _____

Directions: Write one, two, or three aspects of your life you would like to balance from My On-Track Action Plan (Worksheet 3) in the circles below. List several On-Track Actions that will help you actively balance each aspect.

Aspects to Balance   **On-Track Actions**

From *The Emotion Regulation Skills System Workbook, Second Edition*. Copyright © 2026 Julie F. Brown. Published by The Guilford Press. Permission to photocopy this material or download it from the epdf is granted to purchasers of this book for personal use; see copyright page for details.

| LEARNING SKILLS, ON-TRACK ACTION | HANDOUT 6 |

Accepting the Situation

When do I practice acceptance?

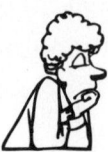 When I have done all I can and have to wait for the situation to change.

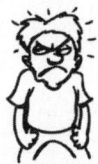 When I have to move away from something because it is making my feelings level go up too high.

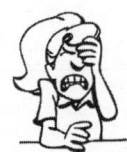 When I have to give my feelings time to go down to or below a Level 3 until I can use my Calm-Only skills.

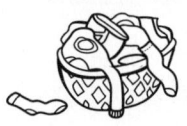 When there are things I don't want to do and have to anyway.

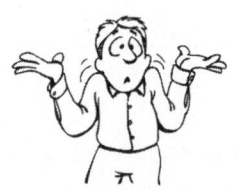 When there is nothing I can do to change the situation right now.

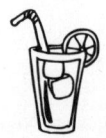 When life gives me lemons, I accept and make lemonade.

From *The Emotion Regulation Skills System Workbook, Second Edition.* Copyright © 2026 Julie F. Brown. Published by The Guilford Press. Permission to photocopy this material or download it from the epdf is granted to purchasers of this book for personal use; see copyright page for details.

LEARNING SKILLS, ON-TRACK ACTION

HANDOUT 7

 Turn the Page

I can get stuck in . . .

- Worries
- Memories
- Painful Emotions
- Off-Track Urges

or I can . . .

- Get a Clear Picture
- Use Lots of On-Track Thinking
- Take an On-Track Action
- Do New-Me Activities to Help Me Focus on the Present Moment
- Have Both Feet On-Track
- Focus on a New Page

From *The Emotion Regulation Skills System Workbook, Second Edition.* Copyright © 2026 Julie F. Brown. Published by The Guilford Press. Permission to photocopy this material or download it from the epdf is granted to purchasers of this book for personal use; see copyright page for details.

LEARNING SKILLS, ON-TRACK ACTION WORKED EXAMPLE 5

Accept the Situation and Turn the Page

Name: _____ Date: _____

Directions: If you would like to sort through whether it may make sense to Accept the Situation and/or Turn the Page, briefly describe the situation and answer the following questions.

Challenging Situation: _I don't like my job. My boss yells at people a lot._

Clear Picture: How do you notice this situation affects you right now?
 Breath: _Fast and shallow._
 Surroundings: _At home after work._
 Body Check: _I have a headache._
 Label and Rate Feelings: _Frustrated_   0–1–2–(3)–4–5
 Thoughts: _My boss stresses me out._
 Urges: _I want to quit my job._

On-Track Thinking: Is acting on that urge on-track or off-track for you? 👍 or (👎)
 What will happen if I act on that urge? _Can't pay my bills._
  I have to get another job before quitting.
 Is it possible to change this situation right now?   Yes or (No)
 Can this situation change in the future?   (Yes) or No
 Will focusing on and talking about this situation right now help the situation get better?   Yes or (No)
 How will focusing on and talking about this situation right now affect your feeling?   (Up) or Down
 Do you want your feelings to go up or down right now?   Up or (Down)

On-Track Action: Describe any On-Track Actions that could help you right now.
 First step to your goal: _Go take a shower to relax._
 Switch Tracks: _Chill out rather than stress out._
 On-Track Action Plan: _Cook a healthy dinner._
 Accept the Situation: _I can't change this tonight._
 Turn the Page: _I will focus on things that make me feel good tonight._

What On-Track Thinking will help you accept this challenging situation for now?
It is too late to look for jobs tonight. I will deal with this tomorrow.

What other skills would help you deal with this challenging situation right now?
I need to do lots of New-Me Activities.

From *The Emotion Regulation Skills System Workbook, Second Edition*. Copyright © 2026 Julie F. Brown. Published by The Guilford Press. Permission to photocopy this material or download it from the epdf is granted to purchasers of this book for personal use; see copyright page for details.

LEARNING SKILLS, ON-TRACK ACTION   **WORKSHEET 6**

Accept the Situation and Turn the Page

Name: _____ Date: _____

Directions: If you would like to sort through whether it may make sense to Accept the Situation and/or Turn the Page, briefly describe the situation and answer the following questions.

Challenging Situation: _____

Clear Picture: How do you notice this situation affects you right now?
    Breath: _____
    Surroundings: _____
    Body Check: _____
    Label and Rate Feelings: _____ 0-1-2-3-4-5 _____
    Thoughts: _____
    Urges: _____

On-Track Thinking: Is acting on that urge on-track or off-track for you? 👍 or 👎
    What will happen if I act on that urge? _____
    _____

    Is it possible to change this situation right now? Yes or No
    Can this situation change in the future? Yes or No
    Will focusing on and talking about this situation right now help the situation get better? Yes or No
    How will focusing on and talking about this situation right now affect your feeling? Up or Down
    Do you want your feelings to go up or down right now? Up or Down

On-Track Action: Describe any On-Track Actions that could help you right now.
    First step to your goal: _____
    Switch Tracks: _____
    On-Track Action Plan: _____
    Accept the Situation: _____
    Turn the Page: _____

What On-Track Thinking will help you accept this challenging situation for now?
_____

What other skills would help you deal with this challenging situation right now?
_____

From *The Emotion Regulation Skills System Workbook, Second Edition*. Copyright © 2026 Julie F. Brown. Published by The Guilford Press. Permission to photocopy this material or download it from the epdf is granted to purchasers of this book for personal use; see copyright page for details.

| LEARNING SKILLS, ON-TRACK ACTION | **WORKED EXAMPLE 6** |

Examples of On-Track Actions

Name: _____   Date: _____

Please list examples of On-Track Actions.

Take a Step toward My Goal: *Go out for a walk.*

Switch Tracks: *Turn off the TV and put on workout clothes.*

On-Track Action Plan: *Exercise for 30 minutes a day.*

Accept the Situation: *Accept that I need to work out.*

Let Go and Move On: *I can't run, but I can walk.*

4. Safety Plan — *Avoid eating Twinkies and Ring Dings.*

5. New-Me Activity — *Listen to music on the treadmill.*

6. Problem Solving — *Go to the doctor about back pain.*

7. Expressing Myself — *Ask a friend about her workout.*

8. Getting It Right — *Ask a friend to take a walk with me.*

9. Relationship Care — *Talk to my friend about how much fun the walk was.*

From *The Emotion Regulation Skills System Workbook, Second Edition*. Copyright © 2026 Julie F. Brown. Published by The Guilford Press. Permission to photocopy this material or download it from the epdf is granted to purchasers of this book for personal use; see copyright page for details.

LEARNING SKILLS, ON-TRACK ACTION **WORKSHEET 7**

Examples of On-Track Actions

Name: _____   Date: _____

Please list examples of On-Track Actions.

Take a Step toward My Goal: _____

Switch Tracks: _____

On-Track Action Plan: _____

Accept the Situation: _____

Let Go and Move On: _____

    4. Safety Plan _____

    5. New-Me Activity _____

    6. Problem Solving _____

    7. Expressing Myself _____

    8. Getting It Right _____

    9. Relationship Care _____

From *The Emotion Regulation Skills System Workbook, Second Edition*. Copyright © 2026 Julie F. Brown. Published by The Guilford Press. Permission to photocopy this material or download it from the epdf is granted to purchasers of this book for personal use; see copyright page for details.

| LEARNING SKILLS, ON-TRACK ACTION | WORKSHEET 8 |

123 Wise Mind

Name: _____ Date: _____

1. What are the three skills in the 123 chain?

   _____

   _____

2. What are the initials of these three skills? _____

3. Write the initials for these skills:

4. **S**afety **P**lan: _____   5. **N**ew-**M**e **A**ctivity: _____

6. **P**roblem **S**olving: _____   7. **E**xpressing **M**yself: _____

8. **G**etting **I**t **R**ight: _____   9. **R**elationship **C**are: _____

10. Using initials, list the skills in these skills chains:

    1234: _____, _____, _____, _____

    1235: _____, _____, _____, _____

    12345: _____, _____, _____, _____, _____

    1236: _____, _____, _____, _____

    1237: _____, _____, _____, _____

    1238: _____, _____, _____, _____

    1239: _____, _____, _____, _____

From *The Emotion Regulation Skills System Workbook, Second Edition*. Copyright © 2026 Julie F. Brown. Published by The Guilford Press. Permission to photocopy this material or download it from the epdf is granted to purchasers of this book for personal use; see copyright page for details.

Safety Plan

LEARNING SKILLS, SAFETY PLAN — SUMMARY SHEET

Safety Plan

Safety Plan is an All-the-Time skill. That means that I can use Safety Plan when I am at any level of emotion, 0–1–2–3–4–5.

First, I use Clear Picture and On-Track Thinking. If I notice any risks, my On-Track Action may be a Safety Plan. For example, if I am near a certain person that causes me to have stress, problems, or danger, I use a Safety Plan to handle the situation. It is best to do a Safety Plan before there is a bigger problem. If I do take an off-track action, go near risk, or do something dangerous, Safety Plans can help me get back on-track.

The first step in Safety Plan is to get a **Clear Picture of the Risk.** There are Inside Risks, such as off-track Thoughts, Urges, Feelings, and Fantasies (TUFFs). There are also Outside Risks, such as people who are a risk or places or things that are dangerous. I handle Inside and Outside Risks before I do things that are off-track.

Next, I rate Level of Risks as either **Low, Medium,** or **High.**

- In *low-risk* situations the problem is far away or contact may cause **stress.**
- In *medium-risk* situations the danger is in the area or contact may cause **problems.**
- In *high-risk* situations the danger is close or contact may cause serious **damage.**

It is important not to **overrate** or **underrate** risk. **Overrating risk** means that I think that a low-risk situation is high-risk instead. This can cause me to avoid activities that are helpful to do. For example, if I rate my first day of work as a high risk, I will not go and may get fired before I even start. **Underrating risk** means that I rate a high-risk situation as low risk. This can lead me into danger and harm because I stay in the area rather than moving away or leaving.

Once I have a Clear Picture and know if it is low, medium, or high, I think about what kind of Safety Plan is best. There are three Types of Safety Plans: **Thinking, Talking,** and **Writing.**

- A *Thinking Safety Plan* is when I think about how I am going to handle the risk and take an On-Track Action to handle the risk. I usually use Thinking Safety Plans in *low-risk* situations.
- A *Talking Safety Plan* is when I tell someone about the risk. When I tell someone what could happen, what I have the urge to do, or how I am going to handle the risk, it helps me stay on-track in tricky situations. The other person can help me think through my Skills Plans. I usually use Talking Safety Plans in *medium-* and *high-risk* situations.
- A *Written Safety Plan* is when I write down the possible risk and dangers that are happening or may happen in the future. I write down plans to handle the risk in safe ways. Safety Plans can use pictures. I usually use Written Safety Plans in *high-risk* situations or when I know I will be heading into a difficult situation. It helps to review how I will keep myself safe! I can give people who are trying to help me the plan, so that we can be on the same page about what will help me.

There are three Ways to Handle Risk: **Focus on a New-Me Activity, Move Away,** and **Leave the Area.**

- *Focus on a New-Me Activity*: This means that I focus my attention on what I am doing or another New-Me Activity, rather than being distracted by the risk. I only pay enough attention to the risk to be sure I am safe and that the situation is not getting worse. I Focus on a New-Me Activity in a low-risk situation and Move Away or Leave the Area as the risk goes up.
- *Move Away*: This means that I go to a safer area or get distance between myself and the risk. After I move, I Focus on a New-Me Activity. I Move Away in *medium-risk* situations.
- *Leave the Area*: In *high-risk* situations, I need to Leave the Area and go where I cannot hear, see, talk to, or touch the risk (e.g., leave the building). I should go to a safer area and do a New-Me Activity. If I am in the community, it may be helpful to return home. I have to be sure that where I go is not risky. It isn't helpful to leave one risky situation and jump right into another one.

Safety Pickle: A Safety Pickle is when we are in a medium- or high-risk situation and it is not possible to move away or leave. We do the best we can and do Clear Picture, On-Track Thinking, On-Track Actions, and New-Me Activities until we can move or leave.

From *The Emotion Regulation Skills System Workbook, Second Edition.* Copyright © 2026 Julie F. Brown. Published by The Guilford Press. Permission to photocopy this material or download it from the epdf is granted to purchasers of this book for personal use; see copyright page for details.

LEARNING SKILLS, SAFETY PLAN   HANDOUT 1

Inside and Outside Risks

Safety Plans help us handle risks that come from inside and outside of us.

Inside Risks	**Outside Risks**
Thoughts	People
Urges	Places
Feelings	Things
Fantasies	

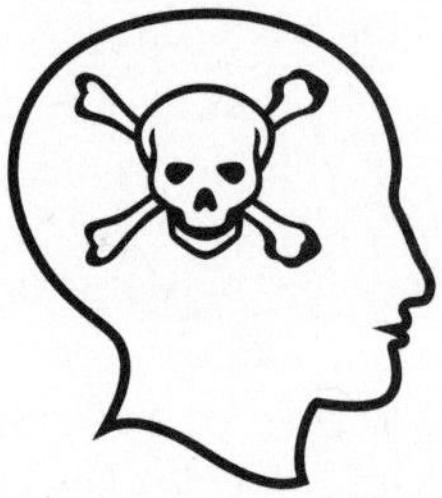

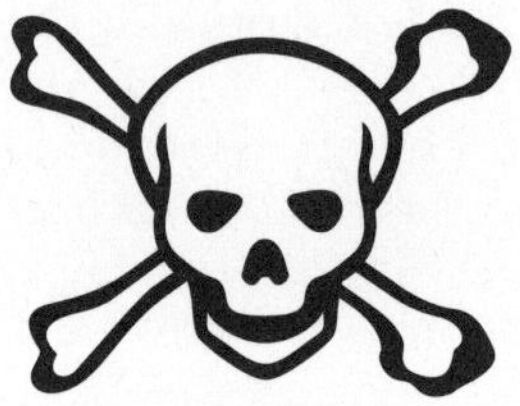

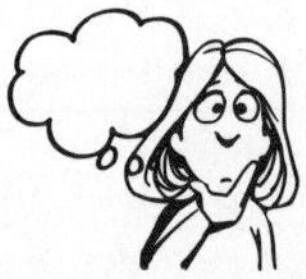

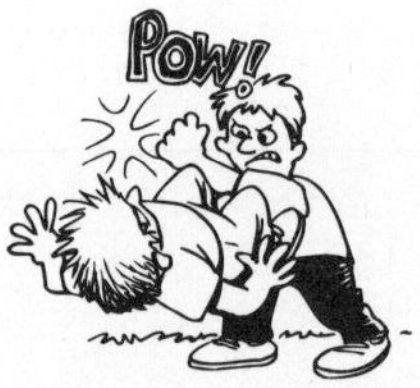

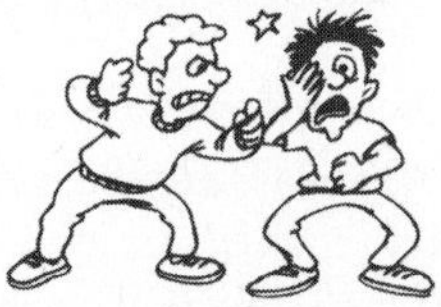

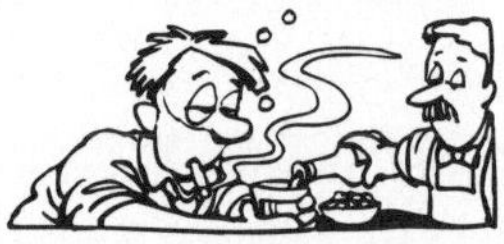

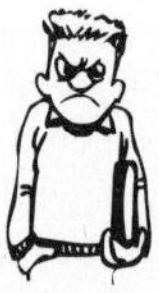

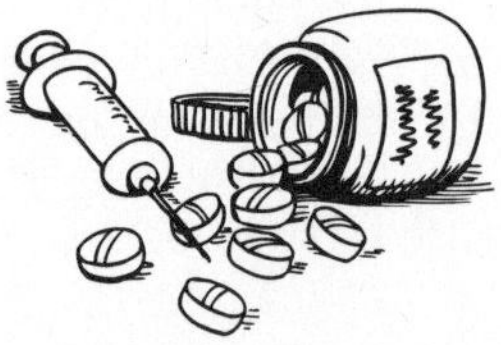

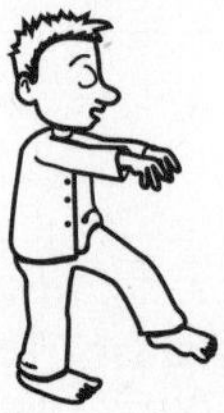

From *The Emotion Regulation Skills System Workbook, Second Edition.* Copyright © 2026 Julie F. Brown. Published by The Guilford Press. Permission to photocopy this material or download it from the epdf is granted to purchasers of this book for personal use; see copyright page for details.

LEARNING SKILLS, SAFETY PLAN **WORKED EXAMPLE 1**

Examples of Inside and Outside Risks

Name: _____ Date: _____

Please list a few of your inside risks.

Thoughts: *He needs to be taught a lesson.*

Urges: *I want to smack him.*

Feelings: *I hate him.*

Fantasies: *I would like to throw him off the bridge.*

List things in your surroundings that are outside risks.

People: *That man stole my girlfriend.*

Places: *The guy who sells me drugs lives on Main St.*

Things: *When I hear "our song," I get mad.*

From *The Emotion Regulation Skills System Workbook, Second Edition.* Copyright © 2026 Julie F. Brown. Published by The Guilford Press. Permission to photocopy this material or download it from the epdf is granted to purchasers of this book for personal use; see copyright page for details.

LEARNING SKILLS, SAFETY PLAN **WORKSHEET 1**

Examples of Inside and Outside Risks

Name: _____ Date: _____

Please list a few of your inside risks.

Thoughts: _____

Urges: _____

Feelings: _____

Fantasies: _____

List things in your surroundings that are outside risks.

People: _____

Places: _____

Things: _____

From *The Emotion Regulation Skills System Workbook, Second Edition.* Copyright © 2026 Julie F. Brown. Published by The Guilford Press. Permission to photocopy this material or download it from the epdf is granted to purchasers of this book for personal use; see copyright page for details.

LEARNING SKILLS, SAFETY PLAN HANDOUT 2

Getting a Clear Picture of the Risk: Three Levels of Risk

HIGH RISK ➡️  Contact with the risk will cause serious damage,

and/or

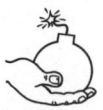 the danger is **close.**

Medium risk ➡️ 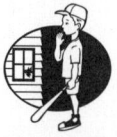 Contact will cause problems,

and/or

the danger is in the area.

Low risk ➡️ Contact will cause stress,

and/or

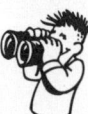 the danger is far away.

Helpful Hints:

Be careful not to rate high risks as low risks.

    This is a problem because I might not Move Away from the risk.

Be careful not to rate low risks as high risks.

    This is a problem because I might avoid a situation when it is more on-track to stay and Focus on a New-Me Activity.

From *The Emotion Regulation Skills System Workbook, Second Edition*. Copyright © 2026 Julie F. Brown. Published by The Guilford Press. Permission to photocopy this material or download it from the epdf is granted to purchasers of this book for personal use; see copyright page for details.

LEARNING SKILLS, SAFETY PLAN **WORKED EXAMPLE 2**

Examples of High, Medium, and Low Risks

Name: _____ Date: _____

Please list your high-, medium-, and low-risk situations.

High-risk situations (close by and/or will cause serious damage)

I am drunk and want to drive.

Medium-risk situations (in the area and/or will cause problems)

I am in a restaurant waiting for a table before dinner and the bartender asks if I want a drink.

Low-risk situations (far away and/or will cause stress)

I am an alcoholic and I hear a beer ad on TV.

From *The Emotion Regulation Skills System Workbook, Second Edition*. Copyright © 2026 Julie F. Brown. Published by The Guilford Press. Permission to photocopy this material or download it from the epdf is granted to purchasers of this book for personal use; see copyright page for details.

LEARNING SKILLS, SAFETY PLAN   **WORKSHEET 2**

Examples of High, Medium, and Low Risks

Name: _____ Date: _____

Please list your high-, medium-, and low-risk situations.

High-risk situations (close by and/or will cause serious damage)

_____
_____
_____
_____

Medium-risk situations (in the area and/or will cause problems)

_____
_____
_____
_____

Low-risk situations (far away and/or will cause stress)

_____
_____
_____
_____

From *The Emotion Regulation Skills System Workbook, Second Edition*. Copyright © 2026 Julie F. Brown. Published by The Guilford Press. Permission to photocopy this material or download it from the epdf is granted to purchasers of this book for personal use; see copyright page for details.

LEARNING SKILLS, SAFETY PLAN HANDOUT 3

Three Types of Safety Plans

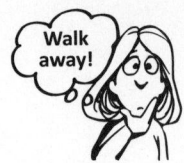 ### Thinking Safety Plans

A Thinking Safety Plan is when I think about how to handle risky situations. I think about whether I should Focus on a New-Me Activity, Move Away, or Leave the Area. Thinking Safety Plans are helpful in low-risk situations.

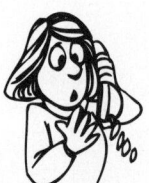 ### Talking Safety Plans

In Talking Safety Plans I talk to someone and let him know about my safety concerns. When I tell him about my risks, he can help me make safe decisions. I talk about whether it is best to Focus on a New-Me Activity, Move Away, or Leave the Area. It is important to be honest and get support in medium- and high-risk situations.

 ### Written Safety Plans

In Written Safety Plans I write down any possible risks that I am concerned about and make a plan to handle each of the risks. In low-risk situations, I plan to Focus on a New-Me Activity. For medium risks, I Move Away, and in high-risk situations, I often Leave the Area. If I think that a situation may be medium or high risk, I may want to do Thinking, Talking, and Written Safety Plans to be sure I will be safe. Written safety plans can have pictures to help me remember my safe places.

From *The Emotion Regulation Skills System Workbook, Second Edition.* Copyright © 2026 Julie F. Brown. Published by The Guilford Press. Permission to photocopy this material or download it from the epdf is granted to purchasers of this book for personal use; see copyright page for details.

LEARNING SKILLS, SAFETY PLAN   HANDOUT 4

Three Ways to Handle Risk

 **Focus on a New-Me Activity in low-risk situations**

In low-risk situations, I can focus my attention on a New-Me Activity. By focusing on what I need to do, I am able to stay on-track AND keep my feelings from going higher. When I stare at the risk, I may become more unsafe and emotional. When I focus on a New-Me Activity, I am able to think more clearly.

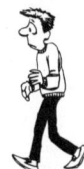 **Move away in medium-risk situations**

In a medium-risk situation, I move away from the risk. For example, if I am having a problem with a person I live with, I should go to my room. Focusing on a New-Me Activity when I get there can help me stay on-track.

  Leave the area in high-risk situations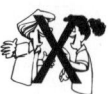

In a high-risk situation, I leave the area or activity. I go to a safer place. It is important to go where I can't hear, see, talk to, or touch the risk. For example, if I am in danger, I may have to leave the building rather than go to another room. Leaving, talking to someone, and focusing on a New-Me Activity in a safe area will help me be on-track.

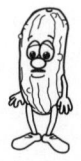 **Safety Pickles**

A Safety Pickle is when I am in a medium- or high-risk situation and I can't move or leave. I use lots of On-Track Thinking and Focus on a New-Me Activity until I can move or leave.

From *The Emotion Regulation Skills System Workbook, Second Edition*. Copyright © 2026 Julie F. Brown. Published by The Guilford Press. Permission to photocopy this material or download it from the epdf is granted to purchasers of this book for personal use; see copyright page for details.

LEARNING SKILLS, SAFETY PLAN **WORKSHEET 3**

Building a Safety Plan

Name: _____ Date: _____

Directions: Please write in a risk. Then circle the type of risk, level of risk, type of Safety Plan (SP), and how you would handle the risk.

	Type of Risk	**Level of Risk**	**Type of SP**	**Handle the Risk**
Risk:	Inside Outside	Low Medium High	Thinking Talking Writing	Focus Move away Leave
Risk:	Inside Outside	Low Medium High	Thinking Talking Writing	Focus Move away Leave
Risk:	Inside Outside	Low Medium High	Thinking Talking Writing	Focus Move away Leave
Risk:	Inside Outside	Low Medium High	Thinking Talking Writing	Focus Move away Leave
Risk:	Inside Outside	Low Medium High	Thinking Talking Writing	Focus Move away Leave

From *The Emotion Regulation Skills System Workbook, Second Edition.* Copyright © 2026 Julie F. Brown. Published by The Guilford Press. Permission to photocopy this material or download it from the epdf is granted to purchasers of this book for personal use; see copyright page for details.

| LEARNING SKILLS, SAFETY PLAN | WORKED EXAMPLE 3 |

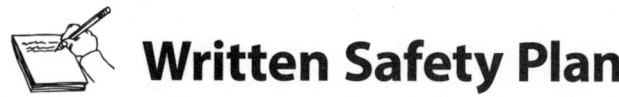 **Written Safety Plan**

Name: _____ Date: _____

Getting a Clear Picture of the risk:

What is the risk? <u> I feel like yelling at my coworker.</u>

Who is involved? <u> Me and Joe</u>

Where is the risk? <u> In the break room</u>

When is the risk happening? <u> 10:00 a.m. tomorrow morning</u>

        Is the risk   LOW   **(MEDIUM)**   HIGH

Making a Safety Plan:

Low risk = focus on New-Me Activities.

    What activity will I focus on? _____

    Who can I talk to? _____

Medium risk = I move away and focus on an activity.

    Where will I go? <u> I will go outside instead.</u>

    Who can I talk to? <u> I will ask my friend to help me.</u>

    What activity will I do? <u> I will take a walk and get some fresh air.</u>

High risk = I leave the area, talk to someone, and do an activity.

    Where will I go? _____

    Who can I talk to? _____

    What activity will I do? _____

From *The Emotion Regulation Skills System Workbook, Second Edition*. Copyright © 2026 Julie F. Brown. Published by The Guilford Press. Permission to photocopy this material or download it from the epdf is granted to purchasers of this book for personal use; see copyright page for details.

LEARNING SKILLS, SAFETY PLAN **WORKSHEET 4**

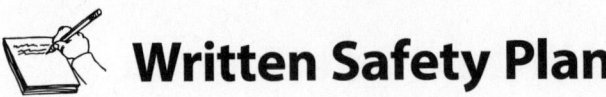 # Written Safety Plan

Name: _____ Date: _____

Getting a Clear Picture of the risk:

What is the risk? _____

Who is involved? _____

Where is the risk? _____

When is the risk happening? _____

        Is the risk   LOW   MEDIUM   HIGH

Making a Safety Plan:

Low risk = focus on New-Me Activities.

What activity will I focus on? _____

Who can I talk to? _____

Medium risk = I move away and focus on an activity.

Where will I go? _____

Who can I talk to? _____

What activity will I do? _____

High risk = I leave the area, talk to someone, and do an activity.

Where will I go? _____

Who can I talk to? _____

What activity will I do? _____

From *The Emotion Regulation Skills System Workbook, Second Edition.* Copyright © 2026 Julie F. Brown. Published by The Guilford Press. Permission to photocopy this material or download it from the epdf is granted to purchasers of this book for personal use; see copyright page for details.

LEARNING SKILLS, SAFETY PLAN — WORKED EXAMPLE 4

Detailed Safety Plan

Name: _____ Date: _____

Directions: Please fill in the sections about the risk. Then check off all the ways that you will handle the risk. At the bottom, list what you will do to be safe. Use the back of this plan as needed.

Risky Event: I got in a fight with my housemate.	**Risky Actions:** I hit him when he took my game.	
	Locations of the Risk: In the living room.	
	Who is involved in the Risk: Me and my housemate.	
Risky Urges:	**Level of Risk:** ☐ Low ☐ Medium ☒ High	**Types of Safety Plans:** (Mark all you need) ☒ Thinking ☒ Talking ☒ Written
	Is There a Safety Pickle: ☐ No, I can move. ☒ Yes, it is difficult to move away.	
Ways to Handle the Risks: ☒ Focus on New-Me Activities. ☒ Ask someone for help.	☒ Move away from the risk. ☐ Remove any risky items. ☒ Leave the house or building.	
Actions I Will Take to be Safe: I will go to safe places: _I will go to my bedroom._ I will avoid: _I will not go near him when I am mad._ I will reach out to: _My brother helps me calm down._ New-Me Activities I will do: _Listen to music with my headphones._ Items I will get rid of: _Anything I could hit him with._		

From *The Emotion Regulation Skills System Workbook, Second Edition.* Copyright © 2026 Julie F. Brown. Published by The Guilford Press. Permission to photocopy this material or download it from the epdf is granted to purchasers of this book for personal use; see copyright page for details.

LEARNING SKILLS, SAFETY PLAN WORKSHEET 5

Detailed Safety Plan

Name: _____ Date: _____

Directions: Please fill in the sections about the risk. Then check off all the ways that you will handle the risk. At the bottom, list what you will do to be safe. Use the back of this plan as needed.

Risky Event:	Risky Actions:	
	Locations of the Risk:	
	Who is involved in the Risk:	
Risky Urges:	**Level of Risk:** ☐ Low ☐ Medium ☐ High	**Types of Safety Plans:** (Mark all you need) ☐ Thinking ☐ Talking ☐ Written
	Is There a Safety Pickle: ☐ No, I can move. ☐ Yes, it is difficult to move away.	
Ways to Handle the Risks: ☐ Focus on New-Me Activities. ☐ Ask someone for help.	☐ Move away from the risk. ☐ Remove any risky items. ☐ Leave the house or building.	
Actions I Will Take to be Safe: I will go to safe places: _____ I will avoid: _____ I will reach out to: _____ New-Me Activities I will do: _____ Items I will get rid of: _____		

From *The Emotion Regulation Skills System Workbook, Second Edition*. Copyright © 2026 Julie F. Brown. Published by The Guilford Press. Permission to photocopy this material or download it from the epdf is granted to purchasers of this book for personal use; see copyright page for details.

New-Me Activities

LEARNING SKILLS, NEW-ME ACTIVITIES — SUMMARY SHEET

New-Me Activities

Solo New-Me Activities are activities we do alone. We can do Solo New-Me Activities at 0–5 feelings. When we do an activity with other people, it is a Partnership New-Me Activity. Because this Partnership involves Relationship Care, we and the other people have to be at 0–3 feelings.

New-Me Activities are the on-track activities that I do during each day. Different New-Me Activities help me in different ways. It is important to choose the right activities at the right time to help me reach my long-term goals. There are four types of New-Me Activities:

- **Focus Activities:** Focus activities improve my attention and focus in the moment. When I do sorting, organizing, following step-by-step instructions, and/or counting, my mind becomes more focused. Examples: solitaire, following a recipe, counting money, folding clothes, cleaning, and playing video games.
- **Feel Good Activities:** I do Feel Good New-Me Activities when I want to soothe myself. I use my senses to enjoy pleasant things. I see, listen to, smell, taste, and feel things that help me feel good. I also may do self-care to feel better. A few examples are walking in a pretty area, using hand lotions that smell good, listening to nice music, drinking a cup of tea, washing my face, taking a bath, and eating chocolate.
- **Distraction Activities:** I do New-Me Activities to *distract my mind* when I want to get my mind on something else (Switch Tracks). A few examples are watching TV and movies, playing video games, and reading. I focus 100% on the New-Me Activity and Turn the Page from the things that are bothering me. I want to be sure I have done all of the other skills I need to before I choose to distract myself. For example, it is often on-track for me to do my chores rather than avoid them by watching TV. Sometimes, though, if I have had a hard day, TV is perfect before my chores. I use Clear Picture and On-Track Thinking to decide what my On-Track Action will be.

I do *distract my body* New-Me Activities when I want to change how my body is feeling. Changing my body can help my feelings and thoughts Switch Tracks. I can distract with cold by holding ice cubes or using an ice pack. I can distract with tastes by eating spicy food or having strong flavored candies or gum (super sour, cinnamon, or minty). I can distract through exercise by doing activities that get my heart pumping and make me sweat. I can walk, jog, run, do yoga, stretch, lift weights, do sit-ups, or use an exercise ball or video to get back or stay on-track. Even though these activities distract me from other things, I have to be focused 100% on the activity. If I am mindless rather than mindful, I could go off-track. It is important that I do these activities in on-track ways to be sure I do not harm myself. For example, ice can burn if I hold it too long, and I can injure myself during a workout if I push my body too far, too fast.

- **Fun Activities:** Fun Activities help me feel happiness and joy. I try to do different things, and that is the spice of life! Examples are drawing, playing sports and video games, working, cooking, cleaning, reading, watching TV, listening to music, talking to friends, going out, studying skills, and so forth. Sometimes I hold back from trying new activities. I do an On-Track Action when I jump in and try something new.

I want to pick New-Me Activities that help me most in the moment. For example:

- If I am getting confused, I choose a Focus New-Me Activity to increase focus and to think more clearly.
- If I am feeling uncomfortable or stressed, I do Feel Good New-Me Activities that help me relax and feel better.
- If I have to wait for a few hours and I want to keep my mind busy, I use a Distraction New-Me Activity.
- If I want to feel good about myself and my life, I do Fun New-Me Activities.

Some New-Me Activities do more than one thing for me. For example, video games may help me focus or distract me from my worries, and they are fun! A phone call to a friend may make me feel good and be fun at the same time.

From *The Emotion Regulation Skills System Workbook, Second Edition.* Copyright © 2026 Julie F. Brown. Published by The Guilford Press. Permission to photocopy this material or download it from the epdf is granted to purchasers of this book for personal use; see copyright page for details.

LEARNING SKILLS, NEW-ME ACTIVITIES   **HANDOUT 1**

Types of New-Me Activities

New-Me Activities are things I do each day that help me to be on-track with myself and my goals. New-Me Activities help me to:

Focus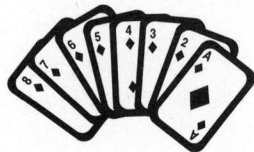

Feel good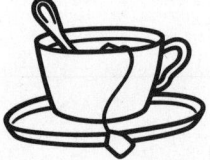

Distract myself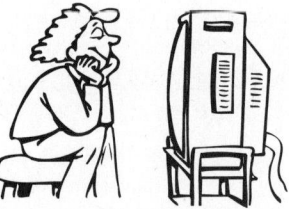

Have **fun**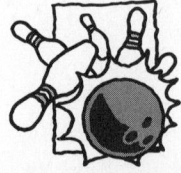

From *The Emotion Regulation Skills System Workbook, Second Edition*. Copyright © 2026 Julie F. Brown. Published by The Guilford Press. Permission to photocopy this material or download it from the epdf is granted to purchasers of this book for personal use; see copyright page for details.

LEARNING SKILLS, NEW-ME ACTIVITIES HANDOUT 2

Solo and Partnership New-Me Activities

SOLO New-Me Activities

Solo New-Me Activities are activities that I do by myself.

I can do Solo New-Me Activities at all levels of feeling 0-1-2-3-4-5.

 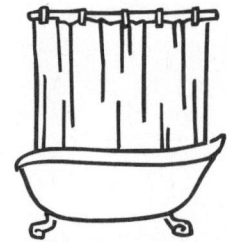 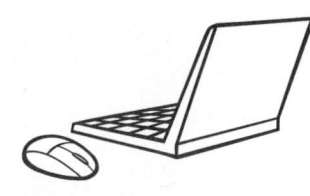 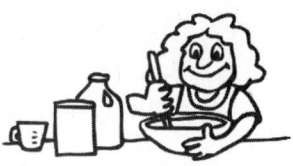

PARTNERSHIP New-Me Activities

Partnership New-Me Activities are activities that I do with other people. Because of this, Partnership New-Me Activities involve Relationship Care. Relationship Care is a Calm-Only skill. This means that I and the other people need to be at 0–3 levels of feelings to do Partnership New-Me Activities together.

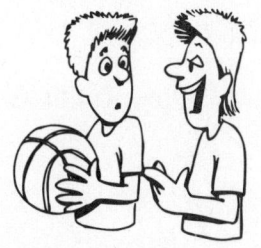 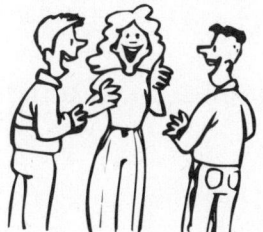 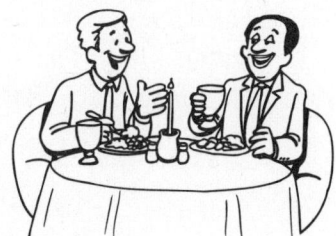 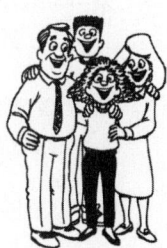

Helpful Hints:

If I am doing a Partnership New-Me Activity and either I or any of the other people go over a Level 3, it may be helpful to get a Clear Picture, do On-Track Thinking, and On-Track Action—Switch Tracks.

From *The Emotion Regulation Skills System Workbook, Second Edition.* Copyright © 2026 Julie F. Brown. Published by The Guilford Press. Permission to photocopy this material or download it from the epdf is granted to purchasers of this book for personal use; see copyright page for details.

LEARNING SKILLS, NEW-ME ACTIVITIES HANDOUT 3

Focus New-Me Activities

Doing Focus New-Me Activities helps me have clear thinking.

They can help me go from feeling

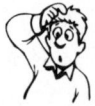 *Confused* to **Focused**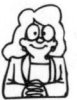

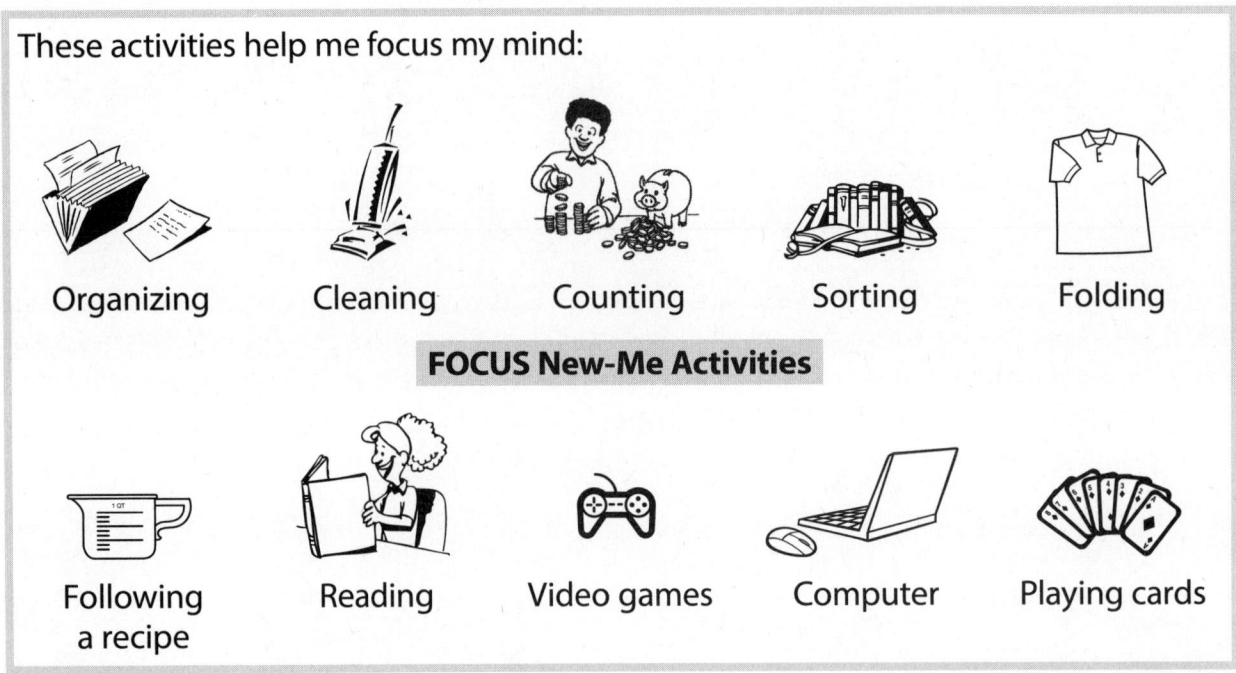

Helpful Hints:

Have a few Solo Focus New-Me Activities to do when feelings are high.

Playing solitaire, doing a word search, making a puzzle, and cleaning help me focus and stay on-track.

From *The Emotion Regulation Skills System Workbook, Second Edition.* Copyright © 2026 Julie F. Brown. Published by The Guilford Press. Permission to photocopy this material or download it from the epdf is granted to purchasers of this book for personal use; see copyright page for details.

LEARNING SKILLS, NEW-ME ACTIVITIES   **WORKSHEET 1**

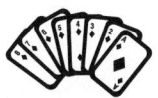 # My Focus New-Me Activities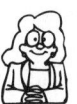

Name: _____   Date: _____

Please list New-Me Activities that help you focus your mind. Check off whether the activity is a Solo and/or Partnership New-Me Activity.

_____   ☐ Solo   ☐ Partnership

_____   ☐ Solo   ☐ Partnership

_____   ☐ Solo   ☐ Partnership

_____   ☐ Solo   ☐ Partnership

_____   ☐ Solo   ☐ Partnership

_____   ☐ Solo   ☐ Partnership

_____   ☐ Solo   ☐ Partnership

_____   ☐ Solo   ☐ Partnership

_____   ☐ Solo   ☐ Partnership

_____   ☐ Solo   ☐ Partnership

_____   ☐ Solo   ☐ Partnership

_____   ☐ Solo   ☐ Partnership

From *The Emotion Regulation Skills System Workbook, Second Edition.* Copyright © 2026 Julie F. Brown. Published by The Guilford Press. Permission to photocopy this material or download it from the epdf is granted to purchasers of this book for personal use; see copyright page for details.

LEARNING SKILLS, NEW-ME ACTIVITIES EXERCISE 1

Body Check as a Focus New-Me Activity

Name: _____ Date: _____

Please sit or lie down. Starting at your feet, tighten and then relax the muscles in each part of your body. This exercise really helps when YOU are at high emotion and want to lower it.

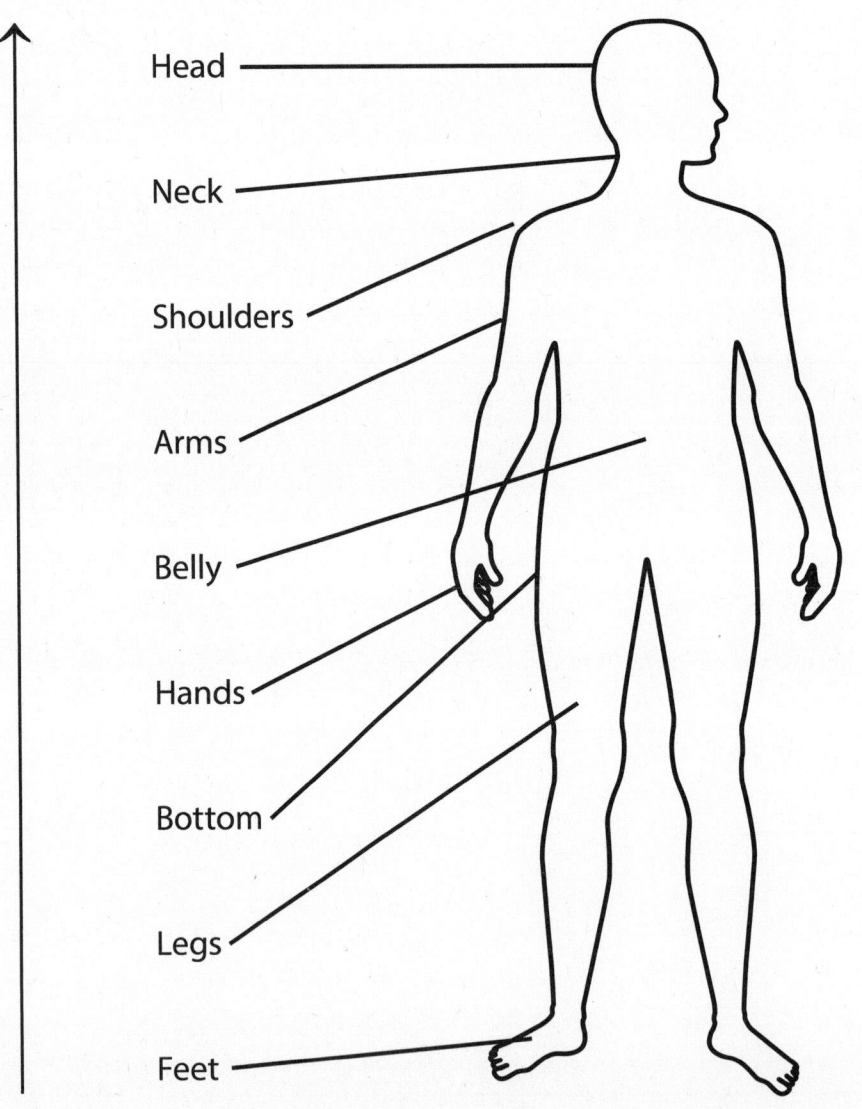

From *The Emotion Regulation Skills System Workbook, Second Edition*. Copyright © 2026 Julie F. Brown. Published by The Guilford Press. Permission to photocopy this material or download it from the epdf is granted to purchasers of this book for personal use; see copyright page for details.

| LEARNING SKILLS, NEW-ME ACTIVITIES | HANDOUT 4 |

Feel Good New-Me Activities

Doing Feel Good New-Me Activities helps me relax and be more comfortable.

They help me go from

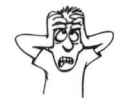 *Feeling stressed* to **Feeling better**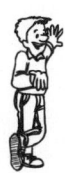

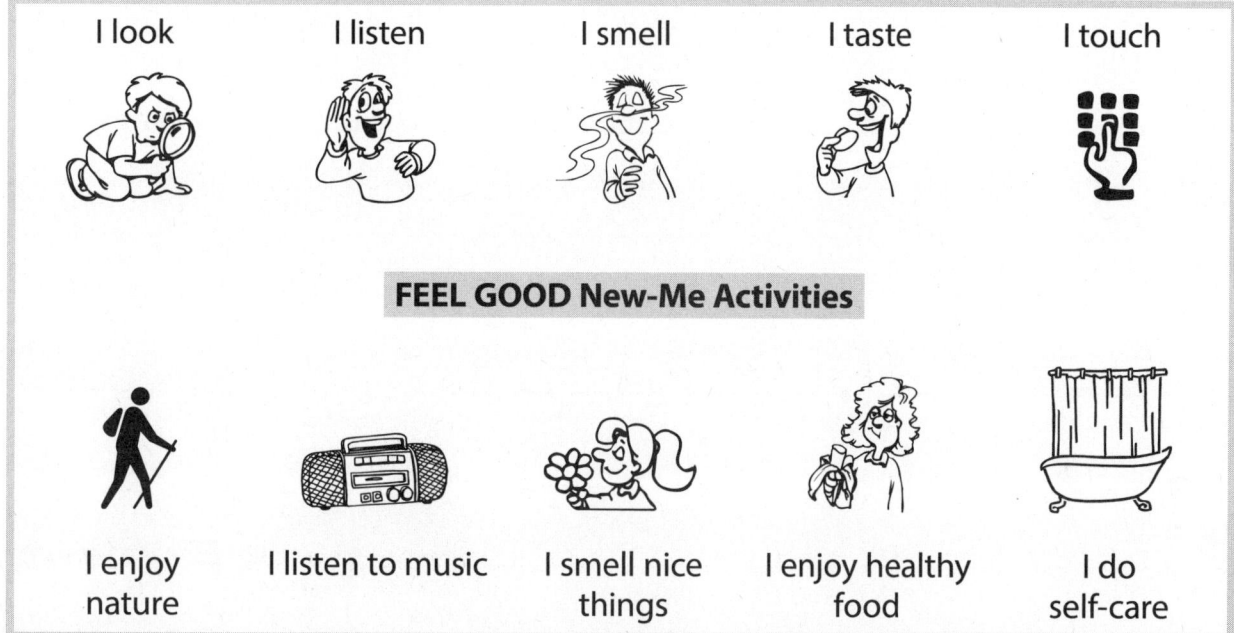

Helpful Hints:

Have a few Solo Feel Good New-Me Activities to do when feelings are high.

Changing into cozy clothes, sitting in the sun, eating chocolate, and belly breathing help me feel better when I am uncomfortable.

LEARNING SKILLS, NEW-ME ACTIVITIES **WORKSHEET 2**

My Feel Good New-Me Activities

Name: _____ Date: _____

Please list New-Me Activities that help your body feel good. Check off whether the activity is a Solo or Partnership New-Me Activity.

_____ ☐ Solo ☐ Partnership

_____ ☐ Solo ☐ Partnership

_____ ☐ Solo ☐ Partnership

_____ ☐ Solo ☐ Partnership

_____ ☐ Solo ☐ Partnership

_____ ☐ Solo ☐ Partnership

_____ ☐ Solo ☐ Partnership

_____ ☐ Solo ☐ Partnership

_____ ☐ Solo ☐ Partnership

_____ ☐ Solo ☐ Partnership

_____ ☐ Solo ☐ Partnership

_____ ☐ Solo ☐ Partnership

From *The Emotion Regulation Skills System Workbook, Second Edition*. Copyright © 2026 Julie F. Brown. Published by The Guilford Press. Permission to photocopy this material or download it from the epdf is granted to purchasers of this book for personal use; see copyright page for details.

LEARNING SKILLS, NEW-ME ACTIVITIES — HANDOUT 5

Distraction New-Me Activities

Doing Distraction New-Me Activities helps me take a break and turn my mind away from off-track things.

They can help me go from feeling

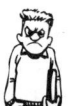 *Frustrated* to **Calmer**

These activities help me distract my mind and my body:

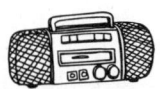 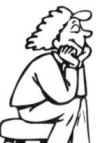 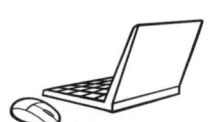 

| Listening to the music and podcasts | Watching TV, sports, and movies | Playing video games or going online | Reading magazines or books |

DISTRACTION New-Me Activities

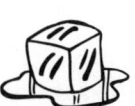 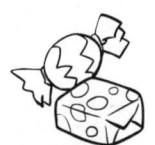 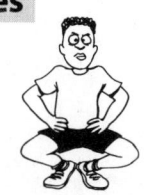

Cold: hold ice cubes/ice packs | Strong flavors: spicy food, sour candy, cinnamon candy, gum, and mints | Exercise large muscles: running, yoga, workout videos, exercise balls, weights, and walking—Do what you can!

Helpful Hints:

Doing Solo Distraction New-Me Activities like watching TV, putting cold water on my face, listening to headphones, and walking outside help distract me while feelings go down.

From *The Emotion Regulation Skills System Workbook, Second Edition*. Copyright © 2026 Julie F. Brown. Published by The Guilford Press. Permission to photocopy this material or download it from the epdf is granted to purchasers of this book for personal use; see copyright page for details.

LEARNING SKILLS, NEW-ME ACTIVITIES   WORKSHEET 3

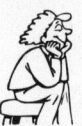 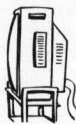

My Distraction New-Me Activities

Name: _____   Date: _____

Please list New-Me Activities that help you get your mind off things. Check off whether the activity is a Solo or Partnership New-Me Activity.

_____ ☐ Solo   ☐ Partnership

_____ ☐ Solo   ☐ Partnership

_____ ☐ Solo   ☐ Partnership

_____ ☐ Solo   ☐ Partnership

_____ ☐ Solo   ☐ Partnership

_____ ☐ Solo   ☐ Partnership

_____ ☐ Solo   ☐ Partnership

_____ ☐ Solo   ☐ Partnership

_____ ☐ Solo   ☐ Partnership

_____ ☐ Solo   ☐ Partnership

_____ ☐ Solo   ☐ Partnership

_____ ☐ Solo   ☐ Partnership

_____ ☐ Solo   ☐ Partnership

From *The Emotion Regulation Skills System Workbook, Second Edition*. Copyright © 2026 Julie F. Brown. Published by The Guilford Press. Permission to photocopy this material or download it from the epdf is granted to purchasers of this book for personal use; see copyright page for details.

| LEARNING SKILLS, NEW-ME ACTIVITIES | HANDOUT 6 |

Fun New-Me Activities

Doing Fun New-Me Activities can add joy and happiness to my life!
They can help turn my mood from

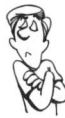 *Grumpy* to **Happy**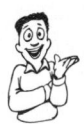

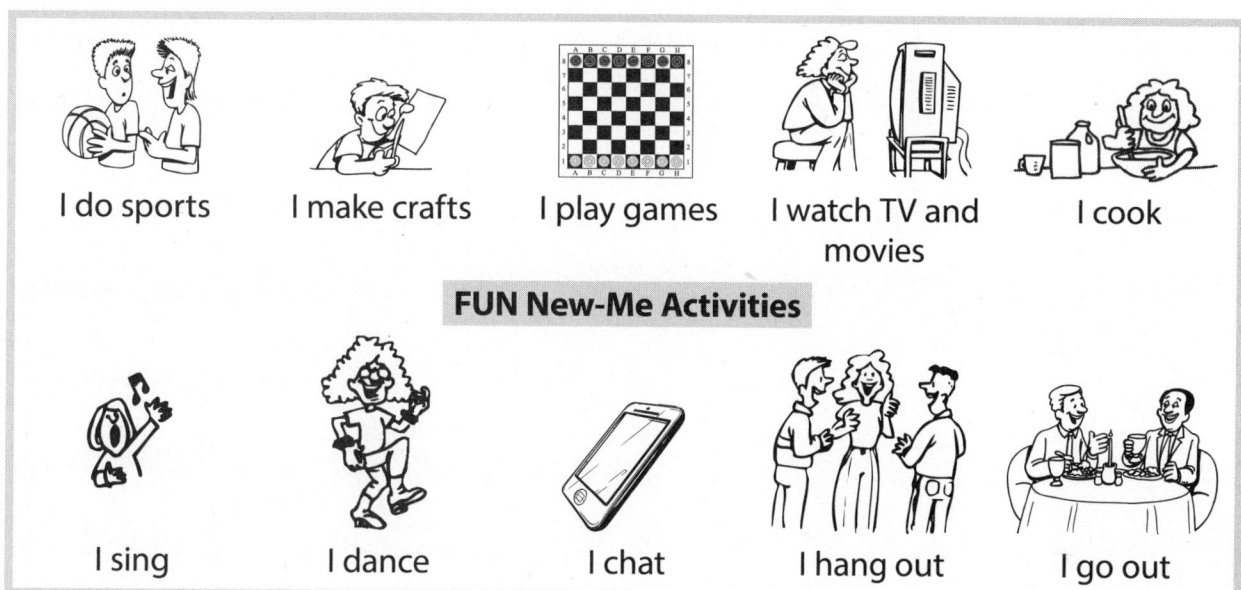

Helpful Hints:

Do Fun New-Me Activities each day.

　　I go to the park, call friends, watch TV, or drink tea.

Have Fun activities that are free and easy to do.

　　I take a walk, listen to the radio, or pet my neighbor's dog.

Try new Fun New-Me Activities.

　　I sometimes need to do an On-Track Action to try new activities. I get nervous at first but then jump in with both feet! Maybe I go to the library, take a bus somewhere new, or go on a picnic.

| LEARNING SKILLS, NEW-ME ACTIVITIES | WORSHEET 4 |

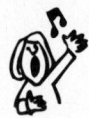 # My Fun New-Me Activities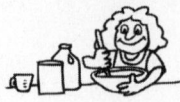

Name: _____ Date: _____

Please list New-Me Activities that help you have fun! Check off whether the activity is a Solo or Partnership New-Me Activity.

_____ ☐ Solo ☐ Partnership

_____ ☐ Solo ☐ Partnership

_____ ☐ Solo ☐ Partnership

_____ ☐ Solo ☐ Partnership

_____ ☐ Solo ☐ Partnership

_____ ☐ Solo ☐ Partnership

_____ ☐ Solo ☐ Partnership

_____ ☐ Solo ☐ Partnership

_____ ☐ Solo ☐ Partnership

_____ ☐ Solo ☐ Partnership

_____ ☐ Solo ☐ Partnership

_____ ☐ Solo ☐ Partnership

_____ ☐ Solo ☐ Partnership

From *The Emotion Regulation Skills System Workbook, Second Edition*. Copyright © 2026 Julie F. Brown. Published by The Guilford Press. Permission to photocopy this material or download it from the epdf is granted to purchasers of this book for personal use; see copyright page for details.

LEARNING SKILLS, NEW-ME ACTIVITIES WORKED EXAMPLE 1

Solo New-Me Activities and Self-Care

Directions: It is important that we take care of ourselves each day. We can do Solo New-Me Activities that help us do self-care. List Solo New-Me Activities that you do currently or need to do in the future. Check whether the New-Me Activities also help you focus, feel good, distract, or have fun.

Do my laundry
- ☒ Focus ☐ Feel Good ☐ Distraction ☐ Fun

Take a shower
- ☐ Focus ☒ Feel Good ☐ Distraction ☐ Fun

Clean my room
- ☒ Focus ☐ Feel Good ☐ Distraction ☐ Fun

Do the dishes
- ☒ Focus ☐ Feel Good ☐ Distraction ☐ Fun

Take a walk
- ☐ Focus ☒ Feel Good ☐ Distraction ☒ Fun

Change my sheets
- ☒ Focus ☐ Feel Good ☐ Distraction ☐ Fun

Make a fruit smoothie
- ☒ Focus ☒ Feel Good ☐ Distraction ☒ Fun

Organize my video games
- ☒ Focus ☐ Feel Good ☒ Distraction ☒ Fun

From *The Emotion Regulation Skills System Workbook, Second Edition*. Copyright © 2026 Julie F. Brown. Published by The Guilford Press. Permission to photocopy this material or download it from the epdf is granted to purchasers of this book for personal use; see copyright page for details.

LEARNING SKILLS, NEW-ME ACTIVITIES **WORKSHEET 5**

Solo New-Me Activities and Self-Care

Directions: It is important that we take care of ourselves each day. We can do Solo New-Me Activities that help us do self-care. List Solo New-Me Activities that you do currently or need to do in the future. Check whether the New-Me Activities also help you focus, feel good, distract, or have fun.

_____
☐ Focus　　☐ Feel Good　　☐ Distraction　　☐ Fun

_____
☐ Focus　　☐ Feel Good　　☐ Distraction　　☐ Fun

_____
☐ Focus　　☐ Feel Good　　☐ Distraction　　☐ Fun

_____
☐ Focus　　☐ Feel Good　　☐ Distraction　　☐ Fun

_____
☐ Focus　　☐ Feel Good　　☐ Distraction　　☐ Fun

_____
☐ Focus　　☐ Feel Good　　☐ Distraction　　☐ Fun

_____
☐ Focus　　☐ Feel Good　　☐ Distraction　　☐ Fun

_____
☐ Focus　　☐ Feel Good　　☐ Distraction　　☐ Fun

From *The Emotion Regulation Skills System Workbook, Second Edition.* Copyright © 2026 Julie F. Brown. Published by The Guilford Press. Permission to photocopy this material or download it from the epdf is granted to purchasers of this book for personal use; see copyright page for details.

Problem Solving

LEARNING SKILLS, PROBLEM SOLVING — SUMMARY SHEET

Problem Solving

Problem Solving is a Calm-Only skill. This means that I can use Problem Solving when I am at or below a Level 3 emotion. When I try to do Problem Solving when I am over a Level 3 emotion, I usually make things worse for myself. I fix problems when I am in Wise Mind; I use 1236 to solve problems in on-track ways.

1. When I notice that something is bothering me in my life, I try to get a **Clear Picture of the Problem.** I think about what I want and what is getting in the way of reaching that goal. For example, if I want to go out to dinner and I have no money, that is a problem. When I have a problem, I can handle it in four ways: (1) fix it; (2) not fix it, but change how I think about it so it bothers me less; (3) not fix it, but Accept the Situation as it is; and (4) do none of these and suffer. I use a 1236 skills chain to figure out which of these I want to do. Doing a Quick Fix and Problem Solving helps me change situations and fix problems.

Size of the Problem: There are different size problems. Small problems are often not too serious and cause low-level feelings. For example, I lost my favorite hat. It makes me a Level 2 sad, but it will not really cause other harm. Small problems usually get fixed with a few simple steps and can be solved more quickly; I can spend $15 and buy another hat. I can do a Quick Fix worksheet to help me solve simple problems. Medium-size problems cause higher feelings (Levels 3 and 4) and take more steps and time to fix. For example, I lost my car keys. Now I have to call a taxi, be late for work, miss my meeting, find out how to get a new key, and get a ride to get a new key. Large or overwhelming problems are very serious, for example, if I lost my job or I don't have anywhere to live. Large problems often cause me to have Level 4–5 feelings, may take longer to fix, and change my life in serious ways.

Fuzzy and Clear: It is important to be clear about the size of problem, so I deal with it in an on-track way. I have a **Fuzzy Picture of the Problem** when I *think a small problem is a large one.* Rather than focusing in the present moment and seeing it as it is (Clear Picture of the Problem), I worry about the future, assume that the worst will happen, think I can control things I can't, and drive my feelings level up. My mind and body can react to some nonemergency situations with a 911 response, so using the skills chain 1236 is important to help me be clear. I can also have a fuzzy picture when I *think a medium or large problem is small.* Doing this can make me not do enough to fix the problem. Sometimes it is hard to know how big a problem is when I first notice it. Taking time to Get a Clear Picture of the Problem helps me stay on-track to my goals.

2. Once I have a Clear Picture of the Problem and decide the solution is not clear enough for just a Quick Fix, I **Check All Options.** I think about a few different things I could do to fix the problem. Each option might lead to some helpful and not helpful results for me. When I Check All Options, I *fast-forward* each option to see what will happen if I take that action. I check the fit of each option to see whether the action would be on-track (thumbs up) or off-track (thumbs down) to my goal. With medium and large problems, it may be useful to list out the *pros and cons* of each option. Pros are the possible on-track or helpful results of an action; cons are the not-helpful or off-track results. For example, Option 1—Yell at my boss. Pro: I will feel better. Con: I will get fired. Option 2—Use Getting It Right to get my hours changed. Pro: I might get my hours changed. Con: I will have to be polite to someone I don't like. I choose the option that has the most pros and helps me reach my goals.

3. Next, I make **Plans A, B, and C.** *Plan A* is the plan that I think will work best to fix the problem. I put 100% effort and focus into my plan. I think about all the steps that I need to take. I think about all the people I need to talk to, what I need to say, and how I will say it. I think about all the other skills I need to use to solve the problem.

After I make Plan A, I think about the fact that sometimes Plan A doesn't work. Sometimes I have to be ready to compromise with the person. I make *Plan B* to have a backup plan that will help me get part of the problem solved. Plan B may help me make the situation better, at least for now, until I can figure out another Plan A that will work better.

I realize that even Plan B doesn't work out sometimes, so I need *Plan C*, which is my fallback plan. I might have another tactic to get what I want. I might plan on Accepting the Situation until I can regroup to make another plan. I might plan to do a New-Me Activity to help me stay on-track as plans fall apart. A Safety Plan might be necessary if I am having urges to take my frustration out on other people.

From *The Emotion Regulation Skills System Workbook, Second Edition.* Copyright © 2026 Julie F. Brown. Published by The Guilford Press. Permission to photocopy this material or download it from the epdf is granted to purchasers of this book for personal use; see copyright page for details.

LEARNING SKILLS, PROBLEM SOLVING — WORKED EXAMPLE 1

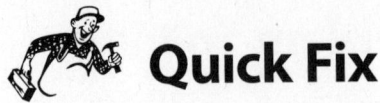
Quick Fix

Name: _____   Date: _____

Directions: Think of a problem and answer the questions.

Problem: _My room is a mess._

What do I want? _My room to be clean._

What is in my way? _Boxes are all over the room._

What is the fix? _Put the boxes away._

What is in the way of the fix? _There are no shelves in the closet._

How big a problem is this? (circle) (**Small**) Medium Large

Now that I have a Clear Picture of the problem, what do I want to do? (circle)

| (**Fix it**) | **Make Lemonade** (Change how I think about the problem) | **Accept the Situation** (Accept it as it is) | **Suffer** (Do nothing different) |

If I choose to fix it, what am I going to do? _Put up shelves in the closet._

What makes the fix difficult? _I don't know how._

Plan: _Ask Jim to help me put up shelves in the closet._
      Use Getting It Right with Jim.

From *The Emotion Regulation Skills System Workbook, Second Edition.* Copyright © 2026 Julie F. Brown. Published by The Guilford Press. Permission to photocopy this material or download it from the epdf is granted to purchasers of this book for personal use; see copyright page for details.

LEARNING SKILLS, PROBLEM SOLVING **WORKSHEET 1**

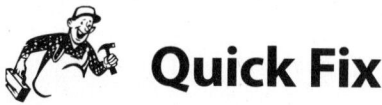

Name: _____   Date: _____

Directions: Think of a problem and answer the questions.

Problem: _____

What do I want? _____

What is in my way? _____

What is the fix? _____

What is in the way of the fix? _____

How big a problem is this? (circle)   Small   Medium   Large

Now that I have a Clear Picture of the problem, what do I want to do? (circle)

| **Fix it** | **Make Lemonade**
(Change how I think
about the problem) | **Accept the Situation**
(Accept it as it is) | **Suffer**
(Do nothing
different) |

If I choose to fix it, what am I going to do? _____
_____

What makes the fix difficult? _____

Plan: _____
_____
_____

From *The Emotion Regulation Skills System Workbook, Second Edition*. Copyright © 2026 Julie F. Brown. Published by The Guilford Press. Permission to photocopy this material or download it from the epdf is granted to purchasers of this book for personal use; see copyright page for details.

LEARNING SKILLS, PROBLEM SOLVING

HANDOUT 1

Problem Solving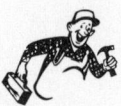

Problem Solving is a Calm-Only skill. I have to be at a 0–3 feeling to do Problem Solving. I have to be focused, so that I can think things through to reach my goals.

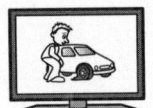 **Clear Picture of the Problem**

What's my goal and what's in my way?

Size of the problem: small, medium, or large.

 Check All Options

Fast-forward each option.

Check the pros and cons.

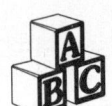 **Make Plans A, B, and C**

Plan A is the best option.

Plan B is a backup or second-favorite option.

Plan C is the option if A and B don't work.

Helpful Hints:

Fix Problems in Wise Mind.

 I want to see small problems as small problems, so I don't overreact and drive my feelings to higher levels. I also want to see big problems as big problems, so I do enough to fix them.

Ignoring problems can make problems bigger and feelings stronger.

LEARNING SKILLS, PROBLEM SOLVING **WORKED EXAMPLE 2A**

🖥 Clear Picture of the Problem

Name: _____ Date: _____

Directions: The first step in Problem Solving is to clarify the problem. As you think of the problem you want to solve, answer the following three questions.

★ What is my goal in the situation?
To get my new sneakers today.
_____

☒ What is keeping me from my goal?
I only have $25 and the ones I want are $75.
_____

🖥 What do I want to fix?
I need to go to the mall to buy new sneakers, and I need $50
more to buy the ones I want.

Size of the problem (circle):   (Small)   Medium   Large

From *The Emotion Regulation Skills System Workbook, Second Edition*. Copyright © 2026 Julie F. Brown. Published by The Guilford Press. Permission to photocopy this material or download it from the epdf is granted to purchasers of this book for personal use; see copyright page for details.

LEARNING SKILLS, PROBLEM SOLVING **WORKSHEET 2A**

🖥 Clear Picture of the Problem

Name: _____ Date: _____

Directions: The first step in Problem Solving is to clarify the problem. As you think of the problem you want to solve, answer the following three questions.

★ What is my goal in the situation?
_____
_____

☒ What is keeping me from my goal?
_____
_____

🖥 What do I want to fix?
_____
_____

Size of the problem (circle):   Small   Medium   Large

From *The Emotion Regulation Skills System Workbook, Second Edition*. Copyright © 2026 Julie F. Brown. Published by The Guilford Press. Permission to photocopy this material or download it from the epdf is granted to purchasers of this book for personal use; see copyright page for details.

LEARNING SKILLS, PROBLEM SOLVING **WORKED EXAMPLE 2B**

👍 Check All Options 👎

Name: _____ Date: _____

Directions: The second step in Problem Solving is to Check All Options. Write down a few options and the pros (thumbs up) and cons (thumbs down) of each option. After weighing the pros and cons, write down the best option at the bottom.

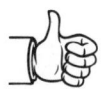 I think of lots of ways to fix my problem and Fast-Forward to see how they will work.

Check the pros 👍 and cons 👎 for each option.

1. _I can steal $50 from work._
   - 👍 Results: _I will get the $50 and my sneakers._
   - 👎 Results: _I will get fired and arrested if I get caught._

2. _I can call my sister to see if she will loan me the money._
   - 👍 Results: _I might not have to pay my sister back._
   - 👎 Results: _She will have to send it, and I won't get the money until next week._

3. _I can save my work money and go next week._
   - 👍 Results: _I should be able to save $50 out of my check._
   - 👎 Results: _I might have to spend the $50 on other things._

4. _I can buy a less expensive pair of sneakers._
   - 👍 Results: _I will get new sneakers today._
   - 👎 Results: _I will not be buying my favorite sneakers._

👍👎 Which is the best fit? _Save my work money._

From *The Emotion Regulation Skills System Workbook, Second Edition*. Copyright © 2026 Julie F. Brown. Published by The Guilford Press. Permission to photocopy this material or download it from the epdf is granted to purchasers of this book for personal use; see copyright page for details.

LEARNING SKILLS, PROBLEM SOLVING WORKSHEET 2B

Check All Options

Name: _____ Date: _____

Directions: The second step in Problem Solving is to Check All Options. Write down a few options and the pros (thumbs up) and cons (thumbs down) of each option. After weighing the pros and cons, write down the best option at the bottom.

I think of lots of ways to fix my problem and Fast-Forward to see how they will work.

Check the pros 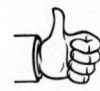 and cons 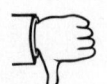 for each option.

1. _____

👍 Results: _____

👎 Results: _____

2. _____

👍 Results: _____

👎 Results: _____

3. _____

👍 Results: _____

👎 Results: _____

4. _____

👍 Results: _____

👎 Results: _____

👍👎 Which is the best fit? _____

From *The Emotion Regulation Skills System Workbook, Second Edition.* Copyright © 2026 Julie F. Brown. Published by The Guilford Press. Permission to photocopy this material or download it from the epdf is granted to purchasers of this book for personal use; see copyright page for details.

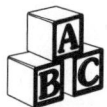 **LEARNING SKILLS, PROBLEM SOLVING**   **WORKED EXAMPLE 2C**

Make Plans A, B, and C ★

Name: _____   Date: _____

Directions: Write down the steps for Plans A, B, and C.

The plan I think will work best is Plan A.

I list the steps I will take to make Plan A work.

A

Plan A: <u>I will save my money and get new sneakers next week.</u>
Steps to Plan A: <u>Next Friday I will cash my check.</u>
<u>I will take the bus to the mall.</u>
<u>I will buy my favorite sneakers.</u>

I make Plan B in case Plan A does not work out.
Plan B is my second-best option.

B

Plan B: <u>If I don't have enough money next week, I will save as much as I can and buy them in 2 weeks.</u>

Just in case Plan A and Plan B do not work, I will make Plan C.
Plan C may be to Make Lemonade out of lemons!

C

Plan C: <u>I will do Problem Solving again in 2 weeks to get new sneakers. I still don't have the money.</u>

🚂 Accept what I can't change.

From *The Emotion Regulation Skills System Workbook, Second Edition*. Copyright © 2026 Julie F. Brown. Published by The Guilford Press. Permission to photocopy this material or download it from the epdf is granted to purchasers of this book for personal use; see copyright page for details.

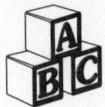 **LEARNING SKILLS, PROBLEM SOLVING** **WORKSHEET 2C**

 Make Plans A, B, and C ★

Name: _____ Date: _____

Directions: Write down the steps for Plans A, B, and C.

The plan I think will work best is Plan A.

I list the steps I will take to make Plan A work.

A

Plan A: _____

Steps to Plan A: _____

_____

_____

I make Plan B in case Plan A does not work out.

Plan B is my second-best option.

B

Plan B: _____

Just in case Plan A and Plan B do not work, I will make Plan C.

Plan C may be to Make Lemonade out of lemons!

C

Plan C: _____

Accept what I can't change.

From *The Emotion Regulation Skills System Workbook, Second Edition.* Copyright © 2026 Julie F. Brown. Published by The Guilford Press. Permission to photocopy this material or download it from the epdf is granted to purchasers of this book for personal use; see copyright page for details.

LEARNING SKILLS, PROBLEM SOLVING — WORKED EXAMPLE 3

Problem Solving Plan

What's wrong: I keep being late for work.
What do I want? I want to keep my job.
What's in my way? I oversleep a lot.
Problem to fix: I have to get to work on time.

Size of the Problem: Small   (Medium)   Large

Check my options to fix the problem:

1. Get my sister to call me at 7 am to wake me up.
   Pros: It will wake me up.
   Cons: She might forget.
2. I can buy an alarm clock.
   Pros: It will wake me up.
   Cons: I might forget to set it.
3. I can ask my boss if I could come in later.
   Pros: I could sleep later.
   Cons: He will probably say "no."
4. I can go to bed earlier.
   Pros: I might get up on time.
   Cons: I probably will still stay up late watching shows.

What option is the best fit? Buy an alarm clock.

Plan A: Get a ride to the mall tonight and buy an alarm clock.

Plan B: Go to bed at 9:30 pm instead of 11 pm.

Plan C: Ask my sister to call me in the morning.

From *The Emotion Regulation Skills System Workbook, Second Edition*. Copyright © 2026 Julie F. Brown. Published by The Guilford Press. Permission to photocopy this material or download it from the epdf is granted to purchasers of this book for personal use; see copyright page for details.

LEARNING SKILLS, PROBLEM SOLVING **WORKSHEET 3**

Problem Solving Plan

What's wrong: _____
What do I want? _____
What's in my way? _____
Problem to fix: _____

       Size of the Problem: Small   Medium   Large

Check my options to fix the problem:

1. _____
   Pros: _____
   Cons: _____

2. _____
   Pros: _____
   Cons: _____

3. _____
   Pros: _____
   Cons: _____

4. _____
   Pros: _____
   Cons: _____

What option is the best fit? _____

Plan A: _____
_____
Plan B: _____
Plan C: _____

From *The Emotion Regulation Skills System Workbook, Second Edition*. Copyright © 2026 Julie F. Brown. Published by The Guilford Press. Permission to photocopy this material or download it from the epdf is granted to purchasers of this book for personal use; see copyright page for details.

Expressing Myself

LEARNING SKILLS, EXPRESSING MYSELF SUMMARY SHEET

Expressing Myself

Expressing Myself is a Calm-Only skill. That means that I can use Expressing Myself best when I am at or below a Level 3 emotion. This also means that I cannot communicate with another person unless he or she is also below a 3. I Express Myself in Wise Mind; I use 1237 to Express Myself in on-track ways.

What is Expressing Myself? When I Express Myself, I share what is *On My Mind* and *In My Heart*. Thoughts, concerns, and needs are a few things that are On My Mind. Feelings, likes, dislikes, hopes, and dreams are a few things that are In My Heart. I Express Myself by talking. I can talk to someone face-to-face, on the phone, through video, and by sign language. I can Express Myself by writing. If I have trouble reading and writing, someone can help me. I can write letters and emails, and I can use social media and texts. Pictures are also a form of communication. I can make drawings and take photos. I can use body language to Express Myself, such as frowning, smiling, eye rolls, sighs, crossed arms, and eye contact. I also Express Myself when I do New-Me Activities. When I sing, dance, play musical instruments, draw, and act, I am Expressing Myself.

Why do I Express Myself? Sharing what is On My Mind and In My Heart can feel great. When I Express Myself through New-Me Activities, it makes me feel better about myself and my life. Doing Clear Picture, On-Track Thinking, On-Track Action, New-Me Activities, and Expressing Myself all together adds joy to my life! I use Expressing Myself with my Calm-Only skills too. Using Expressing Myself, small issues, concerns, and needs don't grow into big problems. I often have to Express Myself when I do Problem Solving to make a situation better. Expressing Myself is an important part of Getting It Right—Right Words (SEALS). I express respect with Sugar. I talk about what I want in Explain. I make a clear request in Ask. I Express Myself to Seal the Deal. Expressing Myself is used in Relationship Care. I feel better about myself when I can communicate and control my life in an on-track way. I talk and listen and give and take in a Two-Way-Street Relationship. I also Express Myself to Find Middle Ground and do Steps of Responsibility when relationships go off-track.

How do I use Expressing Myself? Talking is one way to communicate. There are pros and cons with talking. Some of the pros are that talking can be a quick, easy, and clear way to make a point. The cons are that there can be miscommunication if I don't choose words carefully. Speech and language differences between people can make it more difficult to understand each other. Communicating through writing also has pros and cons. One pro is that when I write, I can make my whole point without interruption. I can also say things that are hard to say face-to-face. I have to be careful not to write things or send pictures I will regret, because the person can look at them over and over again. I am careful not to just communicate with body language. When I try to be a mind reader, or think someone can read my mind, it creates a fuzzy, not clear, picture. Even when I get nervous about Expressing Myself, I do an On-Track Action to share what is On My Mind and In My Heart.

When do I Express Myself? Expressing Myself is a Calm-Only skill. I use Expressing Myself when both the other person and I are at or below a Level 3 feeling. Expressing Myself can make my emotions go higher. Because of this, it may be best if I start expressing when I am at a 0–2 level feeling, so that when I Express Myself and the emotion goes up, I can still be under a Level 3 feeling. If I start at a 3 feeling and it goes up, I will be at a 4! I can't use Calm-Only skills at a Level 4 feeling. When I am over a Level 3, I have urges to Express Myself. I use my Clear Picture, On-Track Thinking, and On-Track Action (123 Wise Mind) to Switch Tracks to a Safety Plan if I go over a Level 3 feeling. Even under a Level 3 feeling, I am careful about venting; it can make my emotions go up. If I want my emotions to go down, I don't vent about things that are annoying me. It can help to talk with a friend to get a Clear Picture of the problem or find a solution, but just venting isn't always helpful if I want my feelings to reduce.

I have to balance Expressing Myself. Overexpressing myself can get my relationship with others out of balance. People's ability to listen to me changes; I may have to ask if this is an OK time to talk. If they say "no," I have to Accept the Situation (or use Finding Middle Ground if it turns into a relationship problem). Otherwise, the person may need to get distance from me. I need to be careful not to underexpress either. This is when I shut down and don't Express Myself when it would be on-track to communicate. Sometimes I am afraid and worry that people won't like me or what I say. I may have to do an On-Track Action—Jump in with Both Feet or Opposite Action—to make myself share what is On My Mind or In My Heart. Do what works!

From *The Emotion Regulation Skills System Workbook, Second Edition*. Copyright © 2026 Julie F. Brown. Published by The Guilford Press. Permission to photocopy this material or download it from the epdf is granted to purchasers of this book for personal use; see copyright page for details.

LEARNING SKILLS, EXPRESSING MYSELF

HANDOUT 1

What Is Expressing Myself?

When I Express Myself, I share things that are
On My Mind and **In My Heart:**

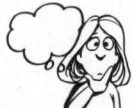	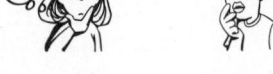	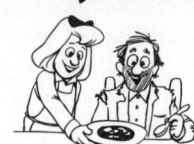	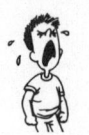	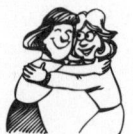	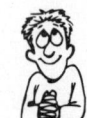
Thoughts	Concerns	Needs	Feelings	Likes and dislikes	Hopes and dreams

Some ways I Express Myself to others:

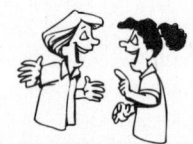		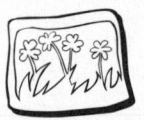	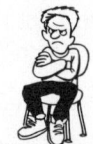
Talking (in person, phone, video, sign language)	Writing (letter, email, texting)	Pictures	Body language

Some ways I Express Myself with myself:

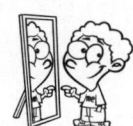	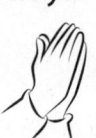	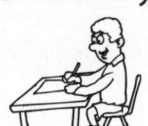	
Talking to myself	Praying	Journaling	Doing art

Some ways I Express Myself through New-Me Activities:

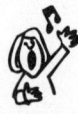	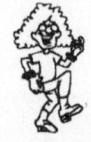	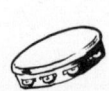	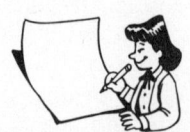	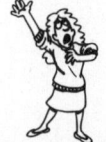
Singing	Dancing	Playing music	Drawing	Acting

From *The Emotion Regulation Skills System Workbook, Second Edition*. Copyright © 2026 Julie F. Brown. Published by The Guilford Press. Permission to photocopy this material or download it from the epdf is granted to purchasers of this book for personal use; see copyright page for details.

LEARNING SKILLS, EXPRESSING MYSELF   WORKED EXAMPLE 1

Expressing What's On My Mind and In My Heart

Name: _____   Date: _____

Please practice expressing as if you were telling someone.

Thoughts: I like watching football more than watching baseball.

I think my cat will need medicine.

Concerns: I am concerned about walking outside at night.

I am concerned I might lose my job.

Needs: I need to have a friend to talk to.

I need to go to the bank.

Feelings: I feel happy that my team won.

I am sad because my cat is sick.

Likes and dislikes: I like pepperoni pizza.

I don't like the taste of raw onions.

Hopes and dreams: I hope to work full time in the future.

Someday I want to buy a car.

From *The Emotion Regulation Skills System Workbook, Second Edition.* Copyright © 2026 Julie F. Brown. Published by The Guilford Press. Permission to photocopy this material or download it from the epdf is granted to purchasers of this book for personal use; see copyright page for details.

LEARNING SKILLS, EXPRESSING MYSELF **WORKSHEET 1**

Expressing What's On My Mind and In My Heart

Name: _____ Date: _____

Please practice expressing as if you were telling someone.

Thoughts: _____
_____

Concerns: _____
_____

Needs: _____
_____

Feelings: _____
_____

Likes and dislikes: _____
_____

Hopes and dreams: _____
_____

From *The Emotion Regulation Skills System Workbook, Second Edition*. Copyright © 2026 Julie F. Brown. Published by The Guilford Press. Permission to photocopy this material or download it from the epdf is granted to purchasers of this book for personal use; see copyright page for details.

LEARNING SKILLS, EXPRESSING MYSELF — HANDOUT 2

Why Do I Express Myself?

Expressing can help me connect to myself and the world around me.

I share what is On My Mind and In My Heart to help me be connected to myself and the world around me. Expressing can help me manage emotions, clarify problems, communicate my needs, and improve my relationships.

Expressing can help me manage my feelings.

Expressing Myself in a balanced way can help me manage my feelings. When I don't express enough, it can decrease my positive feelings. Holding too much in can make me feel worse. When I express too much, it may increase feelings I don't want to get stronger. I use Clear Picture and On-Track Thinking to balance expressing in ways that help me increase the emotions I want to be stronger and decrease emotions I would like to be weaker.

Expressing can help me solve problems.

It can be helpful to share what is On My Mind and In My Heart to help me get a Clear Picture of the problem. As I share about the situation, I can clarify what is happening and how I think and feel about it. If I overexpress and just vent, I may increase my emotions and possibly cloud my vision. I express enough to help me solve problems and not so much that I get a fuzzy picture.

Expressing can help me Get It Right.

Expressing Myself well when I am doing Getting It Right can help me get what I want and need from other people. In Getting It Right I express when I use the Right Words (SEALS). For example, I may want to express respect when I use Sugar. I may want to express thoughts to Explain my feelings about why this is important. I may want to express my requests clearly when I Ask for what I want.

Expressing can help me do Relationship Care.

Expressing things like caring and gratitude can help me build stronger connections and have Two-Way-Street Relationships. Expressing my boundaries helps others know what is OK with me and what is not. There are times when I express and the person responds how I would like, and sometimes they do not. I use Getting It Right and Finding Middle Ground when I want to change my relationships.

From *The Emotion Regulation Skills System Workbook, Second Edition*. Copyright © 2026 Julie F. Brown. Published by The Guilford Press. Permission to photocopy this material or download it from the epdf is granted to purchasers of this book for personal use; see copyright page for details.

LEARNING SKILLS, EXPRESSING MYSELF   **HANDOUT 3**

How Do I Use Expressing Myself?

 Use 1237 to choose how to Express Myself.

There are many ways to Express Myself. When I have something that I want to express, I have to decide how best to express it. I use a 1237 skills chain to decide how to best Express Myself to reach my goals in the situation.

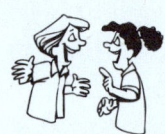 **Talking is one way to Express Myself.**

Talking can be a good way to communicate, but it isn't the only way. It can be a fast, easy, and clear way to make a point. Unfortunately, speech and language differences can make it more challenging to understand each other. Keep trying!

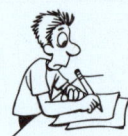 **Writing to Express Myself can be helpful.**

Writing can get my point across in detail and I don't get interrupted. I can also write things that are hard to say face-to-face. Unfortunately, if I write something snarky, the person can read it over and over again. It is helpful to review anything I write to be sure that it is what I want to say and how I want to say it.

 Body language may give a fuzzy picture.

Body language can clarify or confuse messages. A smile, nod, and touch on the arm may communicate caring. Rolling eyes, crossing arms, and fidgeting may communicate disagreement. Body language can add to what I am expressing, so I want to be aware of what my body is communicating. Relying just on body language to communicate may be giving a fuzzy picture.

From *The Emotion Regulation Skills System Workbook, Second Edition*. Copyright © 2026 Julie F. Brown. Published by The Guilford Press. Permission to photocopy this material or download it from the epdf is granted to purchasers of this book for personal use; see copyright page for details.

LEARNING SKILLS, EXPRESSING MYSELF — HANDOUT 4

When Do I Use Expressing Myself?

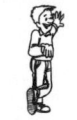
Calm-Only Skill

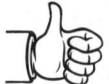 **I Express Myself when it will help.**

I express my feelings, thoughts, likes, dislikes, needs, concerns, hopes, and dreams when it will be helpful for me, another person, or our relationship. If it is not going to help, I wait until I am clear that Expressing Myself is an On-Track Action.

 Start at a 1–2 level because feelings go up!

Expressing Myself can increase feelings. I start Expressing Myself at Level 1 or 2, because when I go into a topic, my feelings can go up. If I start expressing at a Level 3 feeling, it may go up to a Level 4, which is too high for a Calm-Only skill. Doing 1237 helps me know when to stop expressing and Switch Tracks to a Safety Plan and New-Me Activity to help my feelings go down.

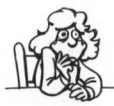 **The difference between waiting and avoiding.**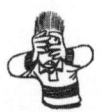

If Expressing Myself drives feelings up, it means that whatever is on my mind could be important. Instead of avoiding it, it may be on-track to wait to express it in a more helpful way. Just waiting until I am calmer may work. Writing a letter or having a friend be with me when I am talking to the person can keep the situation cool. Avoiding expressing important things may make me feel stuck in a bad situation and can drive my feelings higher.

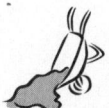 **Be careful of venting.**

Venting with friends about people or situations can feel good, but it actually drives feelings higher. If I want to bring feelings down, I won't vent. If I want them to go up, then I'll vent. Venting can lead to a more negative attitude or it can help me get a clearer picture of the situation. I need to do what works!

From *The Emotion Regulation Skills System Workbook, Second Edition*. Copyright © 2026 Julie F. Brown. Published by The Guilford Press. Permission to photocopy this material or download it from the epdf is granted to purchasers of this book for personal use; see copyright page for details.

LEARNING SKILLS, EXPRESSING MYSELF   **WORKSHEET 2**

Expressing Myself Self-Check

Name: _____ Date: _____

Directions: It can be tricky to know when to express and when not to. When you are deciding whether to use Express Myself, go through this self-check to be sure that Expressing Myself is an On-Track Action at this time.

Expressing Myself increases my level of feelings. It can be best to begin expressing when we are at 0–2 level feelings. If I am at a Level 3 when I begin, there is a chance I will go to a Level 4 when I Express Myself.

    Self-Check Question: Am I between 0 and 2 level feelings? ☐ Yes ☐ No

A Level 3 Sweet Spot is when I am able to have strong feelings, Express Myself openly, AND still talk and listen to the other person.

    Self-Check Question: Am I able to talk and listen? ☐ Yes ☐ No

If I, or the people I am Expressing Myself with, go over a Level 3 feeling, I will be able to Switch Tracks and do All-the-Time skills.

    Self-Check Question: Will I be able to Switch Tracks? ☐ Yes ☐ No

I notice when I am Expressing Myself turns into venting, my uncomfortable feelings go up, when I would like them to go down.

    Self-Check Question: Am I venting? ☐ Yes ☐ No

If I want to change someone's behavior, I will need to use Getting It Right rather than just Expressing Myself.

    Self-Check Question: Do I need to use Getting It Right? ☐ Yes ☐ No

It is important to do Clear Picture and On-Track Thinking to be sure Expressing Myself is an On-Track Action.

    Self-Check Question: Is doing Expressing Myself an On-Track Action? ☐ Yes ☐ No

From *The Emotion Regulation Skills System Workbook, Second Edition.* Copyright © 2026 Julie F. Brown. Published by The Guilford Press. Permission to photocopy this material or download it from the epdf is granted to purchasers of this book for personal use; see copyright page for details.

LEARNING SKILLS, EXPRESSING MYSELF　　**WORKED EXAMPLE 2**

Expressing Myself Plan

Name: _____   Date: _____

What do I want to express?

I want to tell my friend something about her boyfriend.

It is a:　Thought　(Concern)　Need　Feeling　Like/dislike　Hope/dream
Other: _____

Who do I need to Express Myself to?

My friend Carol

Why is it important to express this?

I am worried for her safety.

How can I best Express Myself?

(Talk in person)　Phone call　Video　Sign language　Letter　Email　Text　Body language
Other: _____

When is it best to Express Myself?

I will talk to her Saturday at my house.

Points I need to express:

I care for her and what's best for her.

I heard at work that her boyfriend hit a girl before.

I think she should be careful.

I don't want her to get hurt.

From *The Emotion Regulation Skills System Workbook, Second Edition*. Copyright © 2026 Julie F. Brown. Published by The Guilford Press. Permission to photocopy this material or download it from the epdf is granted to purchasers of this book for personal use; see copyright page for details.

LEARNING SKILLS, EXPRESSING MYSELF **WORKSHEET 3**

Expressing Myself Plan

Name: _____ Date: _____

What do I want to express?
_____

It is a: Thought   Concern   Need   Feeling   Like/dislike   Hope/dream
   Other: _____

Who do I need to Express Myself to?
_____

Why is it important to express this?
_____

How can I best Express Myself?
   Talk in   Phone   Video   Sign   Letter   Email   Text   Body
   person   call   language   language
   Other: _____

When is it best to Express Myself?
_____

Points I need to express:
_____
_____
_____
_____

From *The Emotion Regulation Skills System Workbook, Second Edition.* Copyright © 2026 Julie F. Brown. Published by The Guilford Press. Permission to photocopy this material or download it from the epdf is granted to purchasers of this book for personal use; see copyright page for details.

Getting It Right

LEARNING SKILLS, GETTING IT RIGHT — SUMMARY SHEET

Getting It Right

Getting It Right is a Calm-Only skill. That means that I can use Getting It Right when I am at or below a Level 3 emotion. It also means that the person with whom I do Getting It Right must also be at or below a Level 3 emotion. I use Getting It Right in Wise Mind; I use Skills 1238 to be sure I am Getting It Right in an on-track way.

I use Getting It Right to get things that I want from people.

- First, I make sure I am in the **Right Mind.** I have to be prepared and focused. I have to have a Getting It Right Plan. If my mind is fuzzy instead of clear, I may forget important steps in Getting It Right and not get what I want.
- Then I have to choose the **Right Person** with whom to talk. The right person has the ability to get me what I want. In some situations, I may have to call that person to set up a time to talk. I have to use my other skills, such as On-Track Action and New-Me Activities, while I am waiting to talk to the Right Person. Learning how to wait without losing focus or getting more upset will help me stay on-track to my goal.
- Choosing the **Right Time and Place** is important. I want the person to be able to focus on me, my needs, and how he can help me. Talking to the person when he is too busy lowers my chance of getting what I want. I do what works, so waiting for the best time may increase my chances of being successful.
- Using the **Right Tone** is helpful! I use Clear Picture and On-Track Thinking to decide what tone will work. Usually being wimpy makes the person not take me seriously. Often, being demanding makes him pull away, stop listening, and think that I am not skillful. When I have an aggressive tone, it may stress the relationship so much that the person will never want to help me again, or he will make things more difficult for me. If I notice my tone changing, I need to be sure I am still on-track to my goal. It is often best to step back and wait until another time if I am not able to keep the Right Tone the whole time.
- Finally, I have to use the **Right Words: SEALS**
  - *Sugar*: Using Sugar means I am nice and polite to the person; I make him want to help me. Saying "please," "thank you," and "excuse me, do you have a moment?" makes the person feel like I am giving him respect. I say things that I know will make the person happy about helping me.
  - *Explain the Situation*: I clearly explain why it is important that the person help me. When helping me makes the other person feel good, he is more likely to help me.
  - *Ask for What I Want*: I ask for what I want in a clear and direct way, after using Sugar and Explaining the situation!
  - *Listen*: I listen carefully to what the other person says, so that I can figure out how to Seal a Deal. If he is saying "no," "maybe," or "I don't know," I breathe and focus. If I am going over a Level 3 feeling, it is best to Switch Tracks, stop Getting It Right, and do a Safety Plan.
  - *Seal a Deal*: If the person agrees to help me, then I Seal a Deal and talk about the details. I make sure the person will follow through on what he offered to do. If the person does not agree, I try to either go to Plan B or step back from the situation and rethink the Getting It Right plan.

From *The Emotion Regulation Skills System Workbook, Second Edition.* Copyright © 2026 Julie F. Brown. Published by The Guilford Press. Permission to photocopy this material or download it from the epdf is granted to purchasers of this book for personal use; see copyright page for details.

LEARNING SKILLS, GETTING IT RIGHT HANDOUT 1

Getting What I Want!

We use Getting It Right to get what we want and need from people.

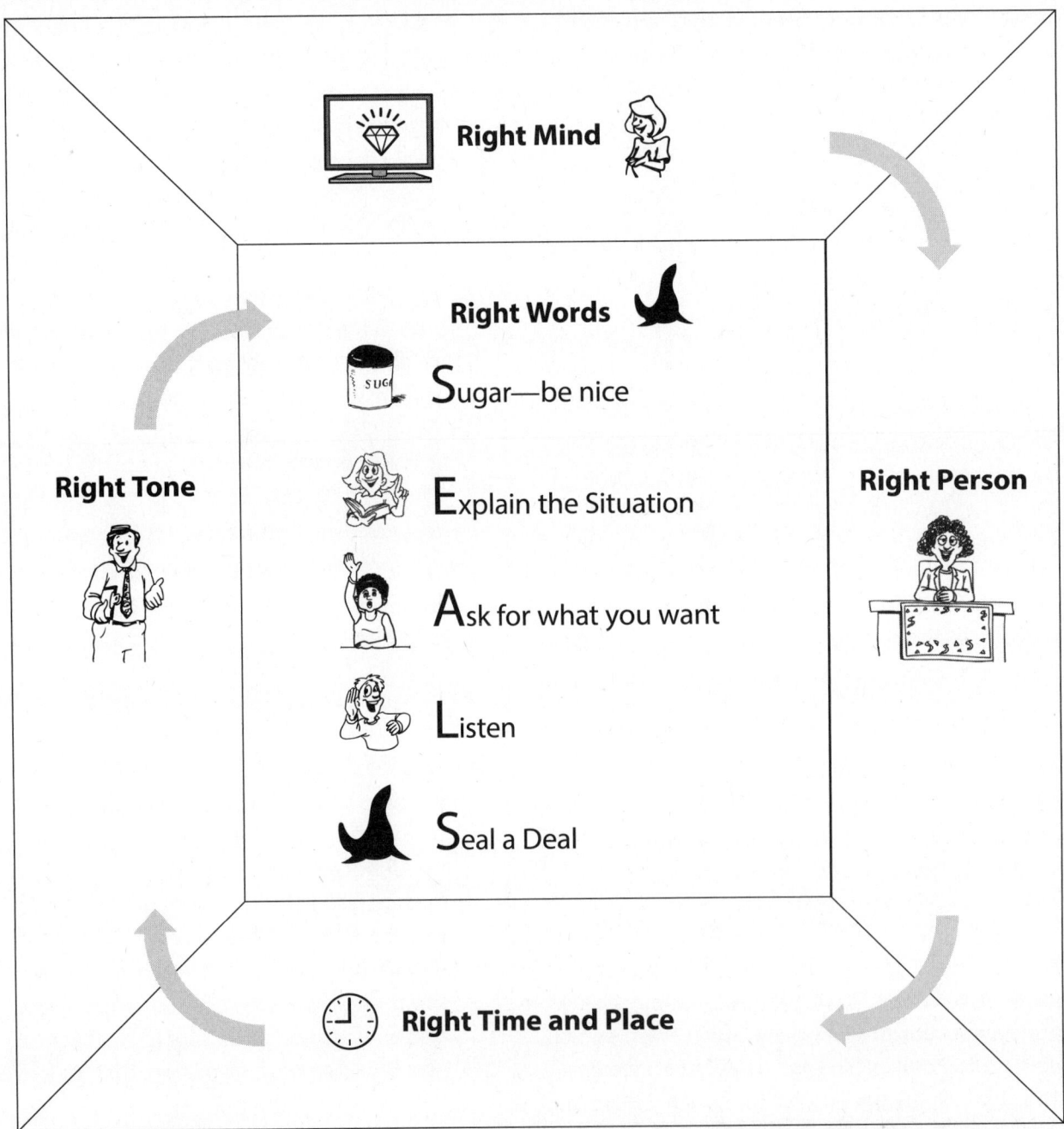

From *The Emotion Regulation Skills System Workbook, Second Edition.* Copyright © 2026 Julie F. Brown. Published by The Guilford Press. Permission to photocopy this material or download it from the epdf is granted to purchasers of this book for personal use; see copyright page for details.

LEARNING SKILLS, GETTING IT RIGHT — HANDOUT 2

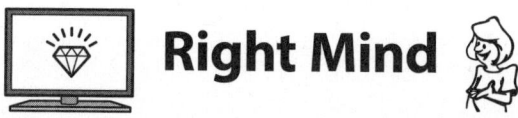

Getting It Right is a Calm-Only skill. This means that I can use Getting It Right when I am at a 0–3 feeling. When I am over a Level 3, I may have strong urges to get what I want—RIGHT NOW. It is hard to get what I want if am scattered and unfocused. Getting It Right takes lots of focus to do well. There are many steps in Getting It Right. I have to wait until I am in the Right Mind to Get It Right!

 **Right Mind means:**

I know what I want.

I am aware of the obstacles to getting it.

I am able to make a Getting It Right plan.

I identify who I need to talk to.

I choose the right time and place.

I think about what tone and words will work best.

I am able to be polite and nice—even if I am a little nervous.

I am able to explain the situation clearly.

I am able to ask for what I want.

I am able to listen to other people.

I am able to work with another person to Seal a Deal.

I am able to DO WHAT WORKS in Wise Mind!

From *The Emotion Regulation Skills System Workbook, Second Edition*. Copyright © 2026 Julie F. Brown. Published by The Guilford Press. Permission to photocopy this material or download it from the epdf is granted to purchasers of this book for personal use; see copyright page for details.

LEARNING SKILLS, GETTING IT RIGHT — WORKSHEET 1

Right Mind Self-Check

Name: _____   Date: _____

Directions: Being in Right Mind is important before and while asking people for anything using Getting It Right. To be sure I am in Right Mind, I will briefly describe what I want and who I need to do Getting It Right with. Next, I will answer the Getting It Right self-check questions to be sure I am in Right Mind before trying to Get It Right.

What do I want? _____

Who am I Getting It Right with? _____

Right Mind Self-Check:

- I know what I want.   ☐ Yes   ☐ No
- I am aware of the obstacles to getting it.   ☐ Yes   ☐ No
- I am able to make a Getting It Right plan.   ☐ Yes   ☐ No
- I identify who I need to talk to.   ☐ Yes   ☐ No
- I choose the right time and place.   ☐ Yes   ☐ No
- I think about what tone and words will work best.   ☐ Yes   ☐ No
- I am able to be polite and nice—even if I am a little nervous.   ☐ Yes   ☐ No
- I am able to explain the situation clearly.   ☐ Yes   ☐ No
- I am able to ask for what I want.   ☐ Yes   ☐ No
- I am able to listen to other people.   ☐ Yes   ☐ No
- I am able to work with another person to Seal a Deal.   ☐ Yes   ☐ No
- I am able to DO WHAT WORKS in Wise Mind!   ☐ Yes   ☐ No

It is important to be in Right Mind before and during Getting It Right.

   Self-Check Question: Am I in Right Mind?   ☐ Yes   ☐ No

From *The Emotion Regulation Skills System Workbook, Second Edition*. Copyright © 2026 Julie F. Brown. Published by The Guilford Press. Permission to photocopy this material or download it from the epdf is granted to purchasers of this book for personal use; see copyright page for details.

| LEARNING SKILLS, GETTING IT RIGHT | HANDOUT 3 |

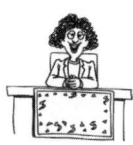 # Right Person

I have to choose the Right Person to talk to when I use Getting It Right. I pick the person who can best get me what I want. It is usually worth waiting to talk to the Right Person. Talking to the wrong person can keep me from getting what I want. Each situation is different; I use Clear Picture and On-Track Thinking to help me choose the Right Person.

The Right Person is usually the person who is in control of what I want:

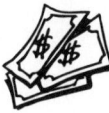 If I want a raise, I usually talk to my boss.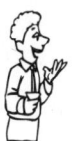

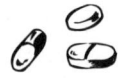 If I want to change my medications, usually I speak to my doctor.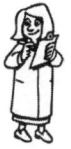

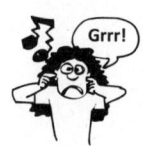 If I want my housemate to turn down her music, usually I speak to my housemate.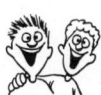

From *The Emotion Regulation Skills System Workbook, Second Edition.* Copyright © 2026 Julie F. Brown. Published by The Guilford Press. Permission to photocopy this material or download it from the epdf is granted to purchasers of this book for personal use; see copyright page for details.

LEARNING SKILLS, GETTING IT RIGHT

HANDOUT 4

 ## Right Time and Place

Choosing the Right Time and Place is important. I want the person to be able to focus on me, my needs, and how she can help me. If the person is busy or distracted, she will not be 100% focused. I want to DO WHAT WORKS so that waiting for the BEST time may increase my chances of being successful. While I am waiting, I need to use my other skills to stay on-track.

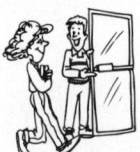 **Choosing the Right Time and Place:**

Speaking to the person in a quiet and private area can help me focus my attention.

I have to be able to focus on using the Right Tone and Right Words.

It may work best if the person is able to focus on what I am saying.

If the person is distracted by something else, it may affect her decisions.

From *The Emotion Regulation Skills System Workbook, Second Edition.* Copyright © 2026 Julie F. Brown. Published by The Guilford Press. Permission to photocopy this material or download it from the epdf is granted to purchasers of this book for personal use; see copyright page for details.

LEARNING SKILLS, GETTING IT RIGHT HANDOUT 5

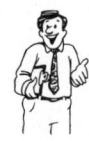 # Right Tone

Using the Right Tone is very important! Each situation is different; I use Clear Picture and On-Track Thinking to decide what tone will work best. Sometimes I want to be gentle; at other times it is best to be firm. I have to think about what tone will make the person hear what I am saying. I want to use a tone that makes the person want to help me.

Choose the Right Tone:

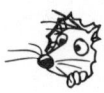 Being timid or passive can make people not take me seriously.

When I have respect and need in my voice,
the person can feel how important the issue is to me.

I respect you.   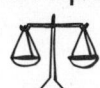   You respect me.

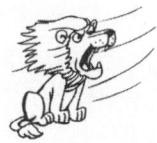 Being demanding can make the person pull away.
Having an aggressive tone can make the person
want to work against me!

From *The Emotion Regulation Skills System Workbook, Second Edition*. Copyright © 2026 Julie F. Brown. Published by The Guilford Press. Permission to photocopy this material or download it from the epdf is granted to purchasers of this book for personal use; see copyright page for details.

LEARNING SKILLS, GETTING IT RIGHT HANDOUT 6

 # Right Words: SEALS

Using the Right Words is important too! I might be nervous when I am Getting It Right, so I plan ahead and practice so that my words come out smoothly.

 I use **S**UGAR to help the person want to help me.

 I **E**XPLAIN THE SITUATION so that the person knows why I need help.

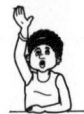 Then I **A**SK FOR WHAT I WANT in a direct and clear way.

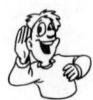 Then I **L**ISTEN carefully so that I clearly understand what the person is saying.

 I **S**EAL A DEAL to get what I want!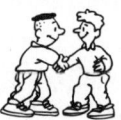

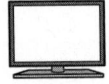 If the person says "no," I do Clear Picture and On-Track Thinking to figure out how to deal with my emotions and get my needs met.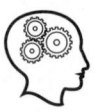

| LEARNING SKILLS, GETTING IT RIGHT | WORKED EXAMPLE 1 |

Getting It Right Plan

Name: _____ Date: _____

Directions: Write down one thing that you want from someone. Fill in all the blanks to create your plan.

What do I want? _I would like more hours at work._

Whom will I talk to? _My boss._

When and where will I talk to this person? _I will ask her to meet. I think we will meet in her office, but I will let her decide._

What kind of tone will I use? _Polite, serious, and like I care._

What will I say to use **S**UGAR? _"Please," "thank you," "I appreciate the time you are taking to meet with me."_

How will I **E**XPLAIN my situation? _I really like my job. I have been here a year and I want to move ahead._

How will I **A**SK for what I want? _I would like to increase my hours._
_____

Will I **L**ISTEN to what the person says?   _X_ Yes   ___ No

What is the deal I want? _I am working 2 days a week now, and I would like to increase to working 3 days per week._

How will I **S**EAL a DEAL? _If "yes," I will ask, "When can I start?" If "no," I will ask, "What do I need to do to increase my hours?"_

From *The Emotion Regulation Skills System Workbook, Second Edition.* Copyright © 2026 Julie F. Brown. Published by The Guilford Press. Permission to photocopy this material or download it from the epdf is granted to purchasers of this book for personal use; see copyright page for details.

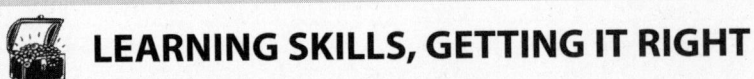 **LEARNING SKILLS, GETTING IT RIGHT** **WORKSHEET 2**

Getting It Right Plan

Name: _____ Date: _____

Directions: Write down one thing that you want from someone. Fill in all the blanks to create your plan.

What do I want? _____

Whom will I talk to? _____

When and where will I talk to this person? _____
_____

What kind of tone will I use? _____

What will I say to use **S**UGAR? _____
_____

How will I **E**XPLAIN my situation? _____
_____

How will I **A**SK for what I want? _____
_____

Will I **L**ISTEN to what the person says? _____ Yes   _____ No

What is the deal I want? _____
_____

How will I **S**EAL a DEAL? _____
_____

From *The Emotion Regulation Skills System Workbook, Second Edition.* Copyright © 2026 Julie F. Brown. Published by The Guilford Press. Permission to photocopy this material or download it from the epdf is granted to purchasers of this book for personal use; see copyright page for details.

Relationship Care

LEARNING SKILLS, RELATIONSHIP CARE

Relationship Care

Relationship Care is a Calm-Only skill. That means that I use Relationship Care when I am at or below a Level 3 feeling. It is also often best if the person I am talking with is below a Level 3 feeling. Building On-Track Relationships, Balancing On-Track Relationships, and Changing Off-Track Relationships are aspects of Relationship Care. I use Relationship Care in Wise Mind; I use Skills 1239 to do it in on-track ways.

I use Relationship Care to Build On-Track Relationships with myself and other people.

An On-Track relationship with myself means that I am getting a stronger Core Self. There are four parts:

1. *Self-Awareness*: I use Clear Picture to be aware of this moment. I see myself and my life *as it is right now*. I also pay attention to my goals and values. When I know what I want and who I want to be, it is much easier to make Skills Plans. Sometimes it is hard to see situations clearly, but in the long run, it helps me stay on-track and feel better about myself. As I learn to see myself clearly, I can see others more clearly as well.

2. *Self-Acceptance*: When I see situations and handle my emotions, it is easier to accept myself and other people. As I interact with others, I see that we are all different and that is OK! That's what makes life interesting! When I notice my thoughts and urges to put myself down, I Turn It to On-Track Thinking instead.

3. *Self-Value*: As I use my skills to reach goals, I get more of what I want. I feel good about my abilities to handle my emotions, my relationships, and my life. I manipulate things in a good way! Doing what works makes me feel better about myself. When I value me, it is easier to value other people.

4. *Self-Trust*: Using my skills, I am able to stay on-track in more challenging situations. I try new things, which makes me happier. I know I can handle anything that comes my way! As I trust myself, I am more able to trust other people. A stronger relationship with myself helps me have better relationships with others.

I use Relationship Care to *Balance My On-Track Relationships* with myself and other people.

—There are many different types of relationships in my life. I use Clear Picture, On-Track Thinking, On-Track Action, and my other skills to make on-track choices to keep all my different relationships in balance.

—Keeping relationships on-track: I take certain On-Track Actions to make the relationship closer when I want to have a stronger connection with someone. I take different On-Track Actions to get distance in the relationship. I use all of these actions to balance my relationships as I, others, and relationships change.

—A *Two-Way-Street relationship* occurs when there is a give-and-take between me and another person. Both of us Talk and Listen, Give and Take. We work together. Respect flows back and forth between us. Two-Way-Street relationships take a lot of attention to keep in balance. Even when I try sometimes, relationships get out of balance. Using other skills such as

LEARNING SKILLS, RELATIONSHIP CARE **SUMMARY SHEET** (page 2 of 2)

Expressing Myself and/or Getting It Right can keep the Two-Way-Street relationship working.

—A *One-Way-Street relationship* occurs when one or the other person is not Talking and Listening, Giving and Taking. Perhaps I feel that I am giving and the other person is not. I may be wanting to have a One-Way-Street relationship if I do not want to Talk and Listen and Give and Take with the person.

I use many skills together to *Change Off-Track Relationships* between myself and other people.

—When I get off-track with myself, I sometimes lose track of my goals, put myself down, and do off-track actions. I get back on-track with myself when I have a Clear Picture of my goals, do On-Track Thinking about myself, and take On-Track Actions. Having and following my On-Track Action Plan helps. Reevaluating myself and my life when I am over a Level 3 might give me a fuzzy picture; it may be best to reflect when at or below a Level 3 feeling to get a clearer picture.

—When my relationship with another person goes off-track, I can use *Finding Middle Ground* and/or *Steps of Responsibility* to get it back on-track.

—*Finding Middle Ground*: First I do Problem Solving to get a Clear Picture of the relationship problem and decide that talking things out is a helpful option. I decide how to Express Myself (e.g., in person, on the phone, or writing). When I do get together (or write), I use Getting It Right to explain my concerns and ask for what I want to change. I listen to the other person's side of the story. We Find Middle Ground when we can find a solution that is good for both of us. I may need to use a 1236789 skills chain to Find Middle Ground! If feelings go up over a Level 3, it is important to Switch Tracks and do a Safety Plan. It may be possible to do Finding Middle Ground at a later time, in a different place, or with other people there to help. When I have tried Finding Middle Ground and serious relationship problems remain, I may have to Accept the Situation as it is, change how I feel about it, or end the off-track relationship.

—*Steps of Responsibility*: When I have done something to hurt another person, I do the Steps of Responsibility. I clearly admit the problem, apologize for what I regret doing, commit to change, and take an On-Track Action that fits for me and makes the relationship better. Taking responsibility can be difficult; I use 1239 to stay on-track.

LEARNING SKILLS, RELATIONSHIP CARE　　　　HANDOUT 1

Building, Balancing, and Changing Relationships

Relationship Care is a Calm-Only skill. This means that I can only use Relationship Care when I and the other person are at a 0–3 level of emotion. When either person is over a 3, we may not be thinking clearly enough to manage relationships well. I use Clear Picture and On-Track Thinking to build, balance, and change my relationships.

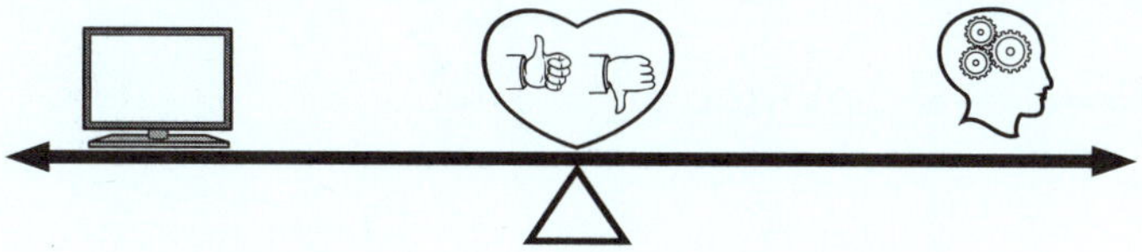

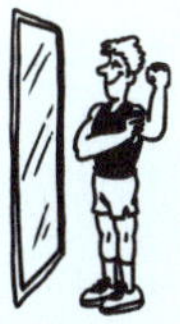

A. Building On-Track Relationships

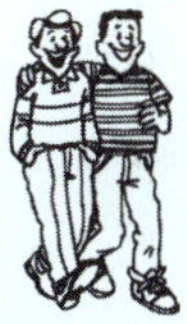

With myself　　　　　　　　　　　　　　　　With others

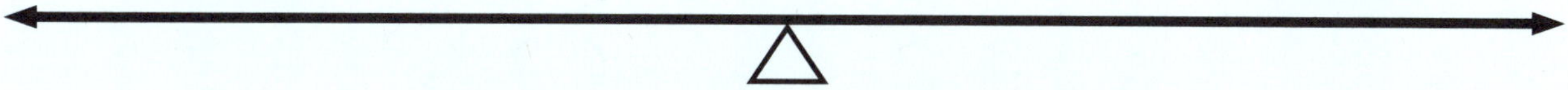

B. Balancing On-Track Relationships

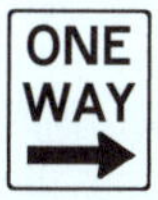

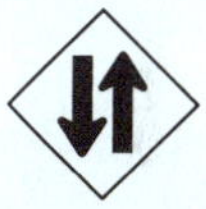

One-Way Street　　　　　　　　　　　　　　Two-Way Street

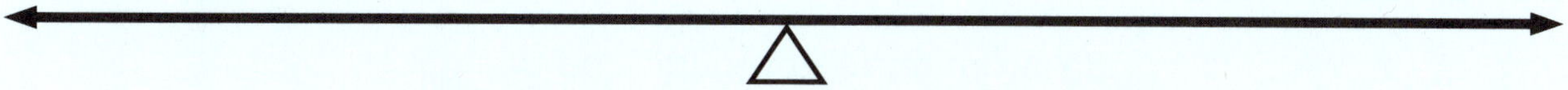

C. Changing Off-Track Relationships

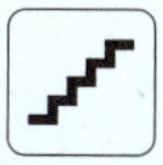

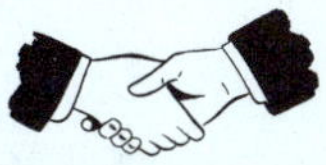

Finding Middle Ground　　　　　　　　　　Steps of Responsibility

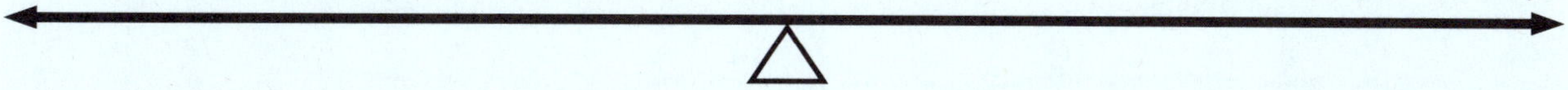

From *The Emotion Regulation Skills System Workbook, Second Edition*. Copyright © 2026 Julie F. Brown. Published by The Guilford Press. Permission to photocopy this material or download it from the epdf is granted to purchasers of this book for personal use; see copyright page for details.

| LEARNING SKILLS, RELATIONSHIP CARE | HANDOUT 2 |

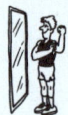 Building On-Track Relationships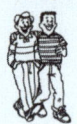

Building an On-Track Relationship with Myself

A stronger core self:

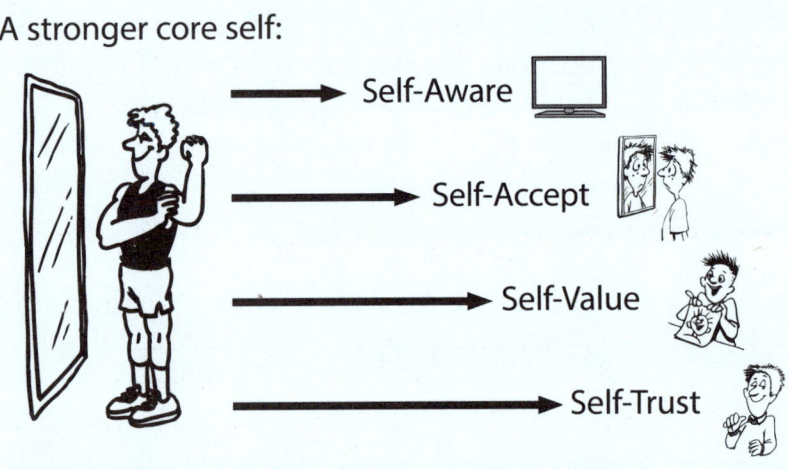

and . . .

Building an On-Track Relationship with Other People

Be aware of, accept, value, and trust

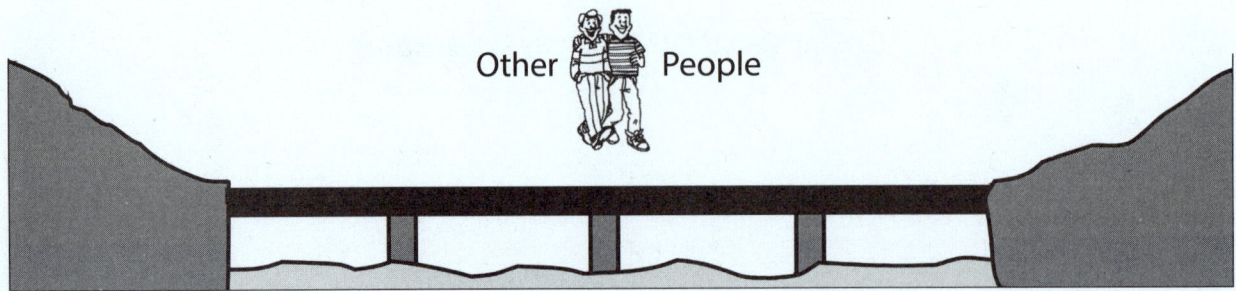

Other People

From *The Emotion Regulation Skills System Workbook, Second Edition*. Copyright © 2026 Julie F. Brown. Published by The Guilford Press. Permission to photocopy this material or download it from the epdf is granted to purchasers of this book for personal use; see copyright page for details.

LEARNING SKILLS, RELATIONSHIP CARE   **WORKSHEET 1**

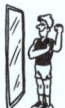 # Building On-Track Relationships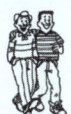

Name: _____ Date: _____

Things I do to build an on-track relationship with myself:

_____
_____
_____
_____
_____
_____
_____

and . . .

How I find new friends and build on-track relationships with them:

_____
_____
_____
_____
_____
_____
_____

From *The Emotion Regulation Skills System Workbook, Second Edition.* Copyright © 2026 Julie F. Brown. Published by The Guilford Press. Permission to photocopy this material or download it from the epdf is granted to purchasers of this book for personal use; see copyright page for details.

LEARNING SKILLS, RELATIONSHIP CARE **HANDOUT 3**

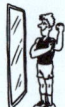 Building On-Track Relationships: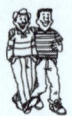
Different Types of Relationships

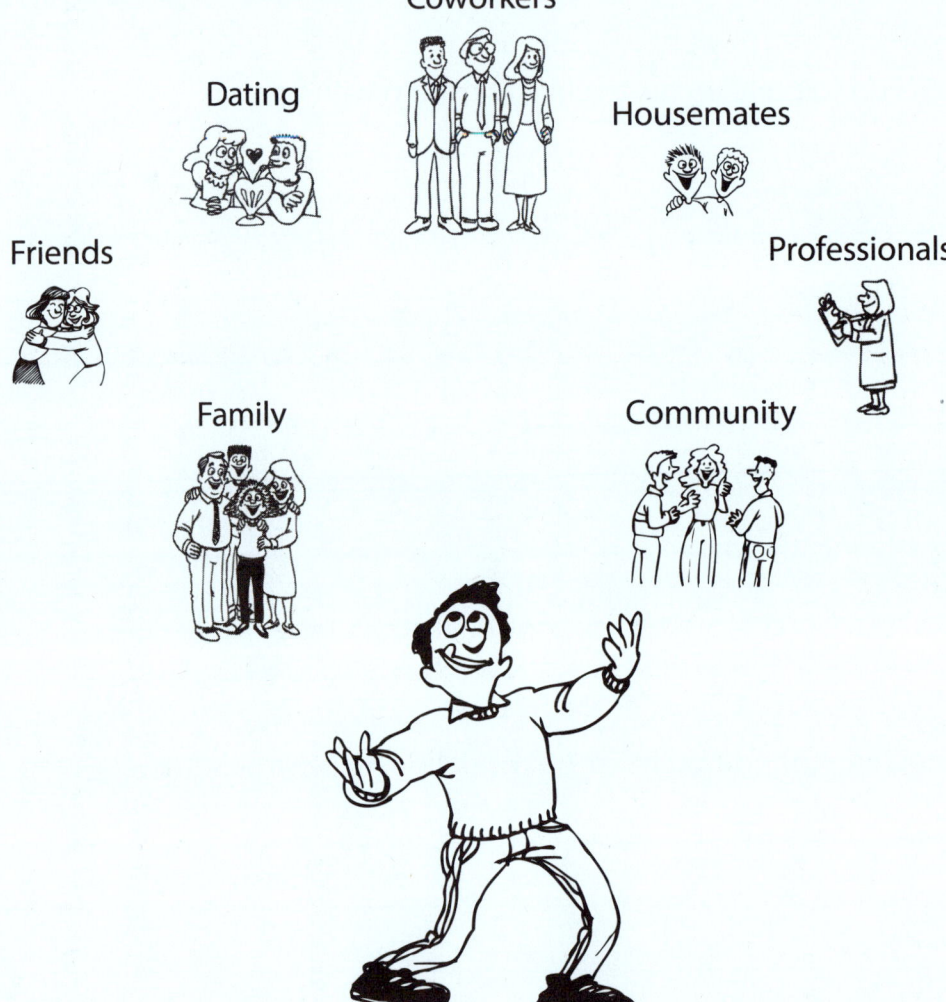

Can you think of others?

LEARNING SKILLS, RELATIONSHIP CARE

HANDOUT 4

Balancing On-Track Relationships

Relationships need a lot of CARE.

Keeping Relationship On-Track

Making a closer relationship ⟷ **Making a more distant relationship**

Closer		More Distant
Act like the person is important.	⟷	Keep conversations short.
Make thoughtful comments.	⟷	Avoid making personal comments.
Call the person/make plans.	⟷	Don't make contact.
Appropriate touch.	⟷	Clear boundaries/keep my space.
Pay compliments/give gifts.	⟷	Focus on what I need to know.
Be flexible.	⟷	Set clear personal limits.

From *The Emotion Regulation Skills System Workbook, Second Edition*. Copyright © 2026 Julie F. Brown. Published by The Guilford Press. Permission to photocopy this material or download it from the epdf is granted to purchasers of this book for personal use; see copyright page for details.

LEARNING SKILLS, RELATIONSHIP CARE   HANDOUT 5

Balancing On-Track Relationships: One- and Two-Way Streets

 In Two-Way-Street relationships, one or both people try to:

 Talk and listen.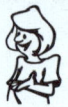

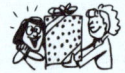 Give and take.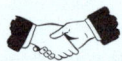

 In One-Way-Street relationships, one or both people are:

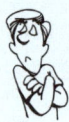 Not listening or talking to each other.

Not giving and taking with each other.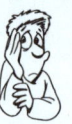

Helpful Hints:

Every relationship is different.

When I have a Two-Way-Street relationship, it is easier to work well with another person.

In a One-Way-Street relationship, it is harder to work together.

Relationships are tricky sometimes!

Even when I try to have Two-Way-Street relationships, sometimes One-Way-Street relationships happen because of me or the other person. I use my skills to care for relationships every day.

From *The Emotion Regulation Skills System Workbook, Second Edition*. Copyright © 2026 Julie F. Brown. Published by The Guilford Press. Permission to photocopy this material or download it from the epdf is granted to purchasers of this book for personal use; see copyright page for details.

LEARNING SKILLS, RELATIONSHIP CARE   **WORKSHEET 2**

Balancing On-Track Relationships

Name: _____ Date: _____

List things that you can do to help make Two-Way-Street relationships.

_____
_____
_____
_____
_____
_____

and . . .

List things you do that may lead to One-Way-Street relationships.

_____
_____
_____
_____
_____
_____

From *The Emotion Regulation Skills System Workbook, Second Edition.* Copyright © 2026 Julie F. Brown. Published by The Guilford Press. Permission to photocopy this material or download it from the epdf is granted to purchasers of this book for personal use; see copyright page for details.

LEARNING SKILLS, RELATIONSHIP CARE   HANDOUT 6

Changing Off-Track Relationships

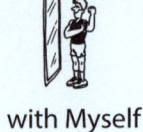

with Myself

Getting On-Track with Myself

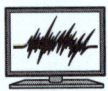 Instead of a fuzzy picture about my goals, I get a Clear Picture of my goals.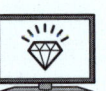

 Instead of putting myself down, I do On-Track Thinking.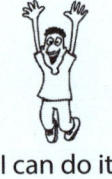

I can do it!

 Instead of off-track habits, I take On-Track Actions to care for my body.

Helpful Hints:

Make an On-Track Action plan.

An On-Track Action plan helps me do things each day that keep me in balance. I don't always follow it, so I have to do On-Track Actions to be sure I jump into New-Me Activities with both feet, use Safety Plans, and move away from situations and habits that are off-track for me.

From *The Emotion Regulation Skills System Workbook, Second Edition*. Copyright © 2026 Julie F. Brown. Published by The Guilford Press. Permission to photocopy this material or download it from the epdf is granted to purchasers of this book for personal use; see copyright page for details.

LEARNING SKILLS, RELATIONSHIP CARE — WORKED EXAMPLE 1

Relationship Check

Name: _____   Date: _____

Directions: Relationship Care can be challenging to manage. We can have relationships with individuals, groups of people, and/or organizations. Relationships can be in balance one day and out of balance the next. If I want to assess whether a relationship is in balance or needs additional care, I will answer the Relationship Check questions below. Getting a clearer picture of the relationship status helps me know if doing Relationship Care would be an On-Track Action.

Name of the person, group, or organization: __Jim—My roommate.__

Clear Picture: How do you notice this relationship affecting you right now?
- Breath: __Heavy__
- Surroundings: __I am talking with my staff now.__
- Body check: __My fists are tight.__
- Label and rate feelings: __Angry__   0 - 1 - 2 -(3)- 4 - 5
- Thoughts: __Jim always takes my stuff.__
- Urges: __Tell him off.__

On-Track Thinking: Is that urge 👍 or 👎?
- Is the relationship a Two-Way street or One-Way street? ⇅ or ➡ ONE WAY
- Would I like the relationship to be different?   ☒ Yes   ☐ No

Making a Skills Plan: Would any of these skills be On-Track Actions?
- ☒ Safety Planning to reduce risks
- ☐ Do Partnership Activities together when at 0–3 feelings
- ☒ Problem Solving—Make Plans A, B, C
- ☐ Express Myself about needs
- ☒ Getting It Right to ask for changes
- ☒ Finding Middle Ground to resolve conflicts
- ☒ Steps of Responsibility
- ☒ Build my Core Self
- ☐ Accept the Situation
- ☐ End the relationship

Other: __Get a locked box__

From *The Emotion Regulation Skills System Workbook, Second Edition.* Copyright © 2026 Julie F. Brown. Published by The Guilford Press. Permission to photocopy this material or download it from the epdf is granted to purchasers of this book for personal use; see copyright page for details.

| LEARNING SKILLS, RELATIONSHIP CARE | WORKSHEET 3 |

Relationship Check

Name: _____ Date: _____

Directions: Relationship Care can be challenging to manage. We can have relationships with individuals, groups of people, and/or organizations. Relationships can be in balance one day and out of balance the next. If I want to assess whether a relationship is in balance or needs additional care, I will answer the Relationship Check questions below. Getting a clearer picture of the relationship status helps me know if doing Relationship Care would be an On-Track Action.

Name of the person, group, or organization: _____
_____

Clear Picture: How do you notice this relationship affecting you right now?

   Breath: _____
   Surroundings: _____
   Body check: _____
   Label and rate feelings: _____ 0 - 1 - 2 - 3 - 4 - 5
   Thoughts: _____
   Urges: _____

On-Track Thinking: Is that urge 👍 or 👎 ?

   Is the relationship a Two-Way street or One-Way street? ⇅ or ➡ ONE WAY
   Would I like the relationship to be different? ☐ Yes ☐ No

Making a Skills Plan: Would any of these skills be On-Track Actions?

☐ Safety Planning to reduce risks
☐ Do Partnership Activities together when at 0–3 feelings
☐ Problem Solving—Make Plans A, B, C
☐ Express Myself about needs
☐ Getting It Right to ask for changes

☐ Finding Middle Ground to resolve conflicts
☐ Steps of Responsibility
☐ Build my Core Self
☐ Accept the Situation
☐ End the relationship

Other: _____

From *The Emotion Regulation Skills System Workbook, Second Edition*. Copyright © 2026 Julie F. Brown. Published by The Guilford Press. Permission to photocopy this material or download it from the epdf is granted to purchasers of this book for personal use; see copyright page for details.

LEARNING SKILLS, RELATIONSHIP CARE HANDOUT 7

Finding Middle Ground

I use all of my Calm-Only skills to change off-track relationships:

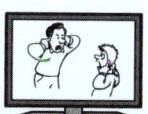
Problem Solving
What is the relationship problem? What are my options? If my best option is to try to work it out, . . .

Expressing Myself
I decide how to communicate: In person? Phone? Email? Letter? Body language?

If I want things to change, . . .

Getting It Right
I choose the Right Time, Place, Tone, and Words:

Sugar

Explain the problem

Ask for change

Listen

Seal the Deal . . .

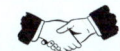
Find Middle Ground
I see both sides and

talk out a win–win solution.

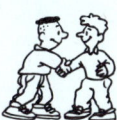

Helpful Hints:

Know when to use a Safety Plan.

If feelings go over a Level 3, a Safety Plan may be a good option.

End off-track relationships.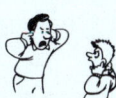

If I have tried to find middle ground and the relationship problems are not better, I may have to end the relationship. I should not be in a situation that is off-track for me.

| LEARNING SKILLS, RELATIONSHIP CARE | WORKED EXAMPLE 2 |

Finding Middle Ground Plan

Name: _____ Date: _____

Directions: If you have a relationship problem, complete the Finding Middle Ground Plan.

What is the relationship problem?
Cindy was rude to my boyfriend.

Planning

How will I communicate: (In person?) Phone? Writing?

Am I in the Right Mind? (YES) or NO

When is the Right Time? _Friday afternoon_

What is the Right Tone? _Friendly but serious_

Should I use **S**ugar? (YES) or NO

How will I **E**xplain my side?
It upsets me when you are rude to my boyfriend.
I am nice to your friends.

To get to know the other side I will ask:
Why don't you like him?

How will I **A**sk for what I want? _Cindy, please be nicer_
to my boyfriend. Talk to me about what is wrong
rather than being rude.

Finding Middle Ground

Will I talk and **L**isten? (YES) or NO

Will I use a Safety Plan if necessary? (YES) or NO

Will I try to find a win–win solution? (YES) or NO

Will I use Skills 123 to help guide my actions? (YES) or NO

From *The Emotion Regulation Skills System Workbook, Second Edition.* Copyright © 2026 Julie F. Brown. Published by The Guilford Press. Permission to photocopy this material or download it from the epdf is granted to purchasers of this book for personal use; see copyright page for details.

LEARNING SKILLS, RELATIONSHIP CARE WORKSHEET 4

Finding Middle Ground Plan

Name: _____   Date: _____

Directions: If you have a relationship problem, complete the Finding Middle Ground Plan.

What is the relationship problem?
_____

Planning
How will I communicate: In person?   Phone?   Writing?
Am I in the Right Mind?   YES   or   NO
When is the Right Time? _____
What is the Right Tone? _____
Should I use **S**ugar?   YES   or   NO

How will I **E**xplain my side? _____
_____
_____

To get to know the other side I will ask: _____
_____

How will I **A**sk for what I want? _____
_____
_____

Finding Middle Ground
Will I talk and **L**isten?   YES   or   NO
Will I use a Safety Plan if necessary?   YES   or   NO
Will I try to find a win–win solution?   YES   or   NO
Will I use Skills 123 to help guide my actions?   YES   or   NO

From *The Emotion Regulation Skills System Workbook, Second Edition.* Copyright © 2026 Julie F. Brown. Published by The Guilford Press. Permission to photocopy this material or download it from the epdf is granted to purchasers of this book for personal use; see copyright page for details.

LEARNING SKILLS, RELATIONSHIP CARE HANDOUT 8

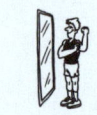 # Changing Off-Track Relationships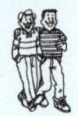

with Myself   and with Others

We do Steps of Responsibility when we have done something to harm a relationship and want to get it back on-track.

Steps of Responsibility

I made a mistake. → **Admit the problem.** → **Apologize.** → **Commit to change.** → **Take an On-Track Action.**

I made a mistake.	Admit the problem.	Apologize.	Commit to change.	Take an On-Track Action.
I said or did something that hurt a relationship that is important to me.	I use Expressing Myself to explain what I did and why it was a problem.	I apologize for what I feel sorry for doing.	If I want to get the other person's trust back, I explain how I will be different in the future.	I take On-Track Actions in the relationship.

Helpful Hints:

Taking responsibility can increase feelings.

Relationships can be confusing. I sometimes don't even know when I have hurt another person. Finding out about my mistakes can make me feel guilty, ashamed, and even angry. I use Clear Picture and lots of On-Track Thinking to be sure that Relationship Care is an On-Track Action at that time. I want to help the relationship rather than make things worse! I do a Safety Plan and stop doing the steps if I go over a Level 3.

From *The Emotion Regulation Skills System Workbook, Second Edition*. Copyright © 2026 Julie F. Brown. Published by The Guilford Press. Permission to photocopy this material or download it from the epdf is granted to purchasers of this book for personal use; see copyright page for details.

LEARNING SKILLS, RELATIONSHIP CARE **WORKED EXAMPLE 3**

Steps of Responsibility

Name: _____ Date: _____

If you have done something you regret and want to get the relationship back on-track, write how you will complete each step.

Admit the problem.

I was rude to your boyfriend.

Apologize for the harm that was done.

I am sorry that I said those things and put you in the middle.

Commit to changing the behavior.

I will talk to you in private next time when I have concerns.

Take an On-Track Action.

I will tell her, "Thanks for being such a good friend."

From *The Emotion Regulation Skills System Workbook, Second Edition*. Copyright © 2026 Julie F. Brown. Published by The Guilford Press. Permission to photocopy this material or download it from the epdf is granted to purchasers of this book for personal use; see copyright page for details.

LEARNING SKILLS, RELATIONSHIP CARE WORKSHEET 5

Steps of Responsibility

Name: _____   Date: _____

If you have done something you regret and want to get the relationship back on-track, write how you will complete each step.

Admit the problem.

_____
_____

Apologize for the harm that was done.

_____
_____

Commit to changing the behavior.

_____
_____

Take an On-Track Action.

_____
_____

From *The Emotion Regulation Skills System Workbook, Second Edition.* Copyright © 2026 Julie F. Brown. Published by The Guilford Press. Permission to photocopy this material or download it from the epdf is granted to purchasers of this book for personal use; see copyright page for details.

Using Skills in My Life

| LEARNING SKILLS, USING SKILLS IN MY LIFE | SKILLS QUIZ |

Using Skills in My Life

Name: _____ Date: _____

1. What skill helps me see the moment? _____

2. What skill do I always use after Clear Picture?
   _____

3. What are the numbers of the three skills I use first in all situations?
   _____, _____, and _____

4. What is the skill I use when I do something positive to step toward my goals?
   _____

5. What skill helps me handle risky situations?
   _____

6. What skill helps me focus, feel better, distract myself, and have fun?
   _____

7. What skill helps me fix situations?
   _____

8. What skill helps me communicate with people?
   _____

9. What skill helps me get what I want from people?
   _____

10. What skill helps me have a positive relationship with myself?
    _____

11. What skill helps me have positive relationships with other people?
    _____

From *The Emotion Regulation Skills System Workbook, Second Edition*. Copyright © 2026 Julie F. Brown. Published by The Guilford Press. Permission to photocopy this material or download it from the epdf is granted to purchasers of this book for personal use; see copyright page for details.

| LEARNING SKILLS, USING SKILLS IN MY LIFE | SKILLS QUIZ ANSWER SHEET |

Using Skills in My Life

Name: _____   Date: _____

1. What skill helps me see the moment? _Clear Picture_

2. What skill do I always use after Clear Picture?
   On-Track Thinking

3. What are the numbers of the three skills I use first in all situations?
   _1_, _2_, and _3_

4. What is the skill I use when I do something positive to step toward my goals?
   On-Track Action

5. What skill helps me handle risky situations?
   Safety Plan

6. What skill helps me focus, feel better, distract myself, and have fun?
   New-Me Activities

7. What skill helps me fix situations?
   Problem Solving

8. What skill helps me communicate with people?
   Expressing Myself

9. What skill helps me get what I want from people?
   Getting It Right

10. What skill helps me have a positive relationship with myself?
    Relationship Care

11. What skill helps me have positive relationships with other people?
    Relationship Care

From *The Emotion Regulation Skills System Workbook, Second Edition*. Copyright © 2026 Julie F. Brown. Published by The Guilford Press. Permission to photocopy this material or download it from the epdf is granted to purchasers of this book for personal use; see copyright page for details.

LEARNING SKILLS, USING SKILLS IN MY LIFE

SKILLS PLAN MAP

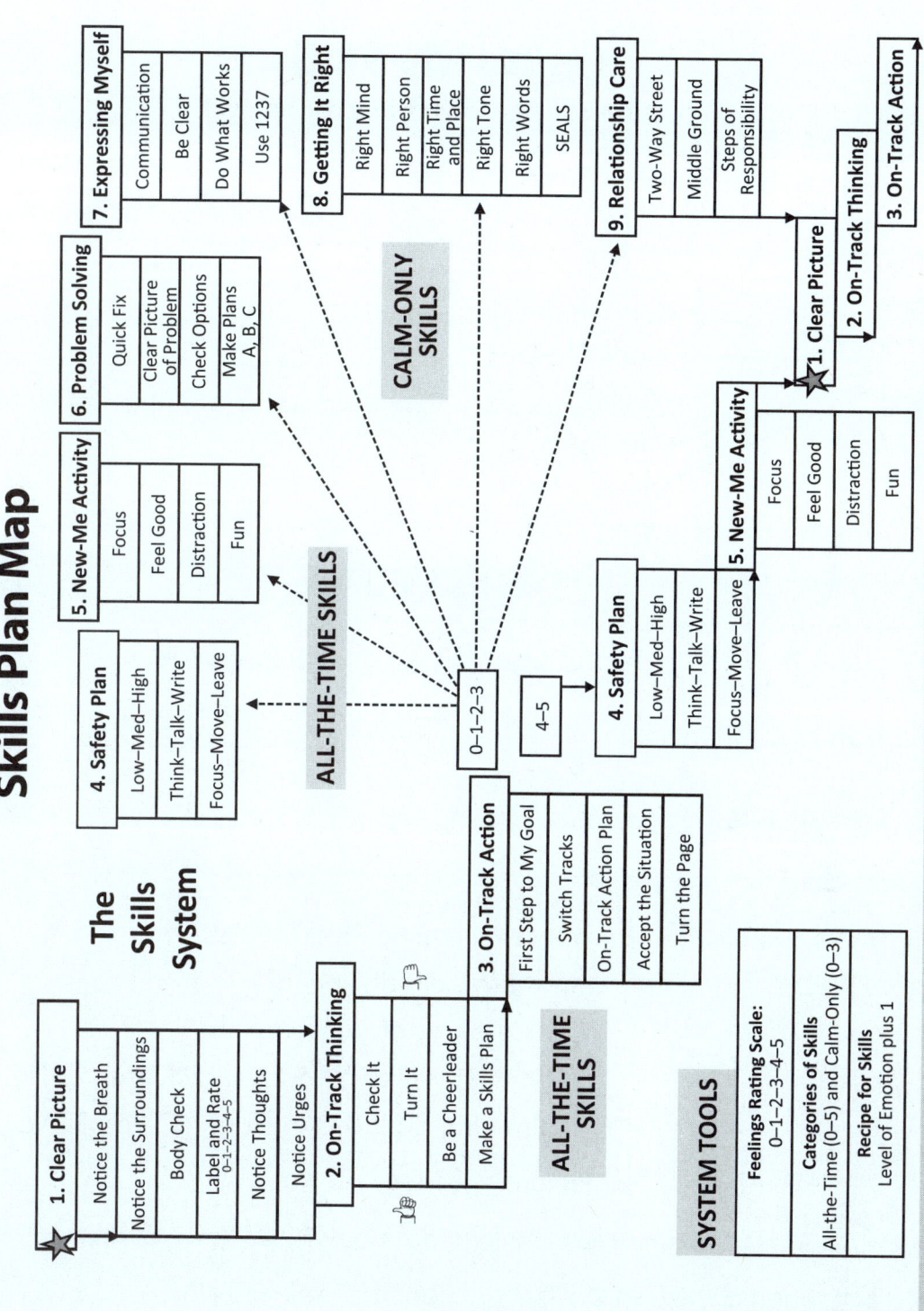

| LEARNING SKILLS, USING SKILLS IN MY LIFE | **WORKSHEET 1** (page 1 of 3) |

Using My Skills
(when at a Level 3 feeling or below)

Name: _____ Date: _____

1. Clear Picture

- Breathe ☐ Yes ☐ No
- Surroundings: _____
- Body Check: _____
- Feeling: _____ Rating: 0–1–2–3–4–5
- Thought: _____
- Urge: _____

2. On-Track Thinking

Check It ☐ 👍 Helpful urge ☐ 👎 Not helpful urge

Turn It 👍 thinking: _____

Cheerleading: _____
_____

Make a Skills Plan: My level of feeling RIGHT NOW: _____

How many skills do I need? _____

What Category of Skills can I use?

All-the-Time skills 0–5 feeling: ☐ Yes ☐ No

Calm-Only skills 0–3 feeling: ☐ Yes ☐ No

Have I used Clear Picture? ☐ Yes ☐ No

Am I using On-Track Thinking right now? ☐ Yes ☐ No

Should I take an On-Track Action? ☐ Yes ☐ No

(continued)

From *The Emotion Regulation Skills System Workbook, Second Edition.* Copyright © 2026 Julie F. Brown. Published by The Guilford Press. Permission to photocopy this material or download it from the epdf is granted to purchasers of this book for personal use; see copyright page for details.

LEARNING SKILLS, USING SKILLS IN MY LIFE

WORKSHEET 1
(page 2 of 3)

Should I use a Safety Plan? Is there any risk?   ☐ Yes   ☐ No
☐ Thinking   ☐ Talking   ☐ Written
☐ Low risk   ☐ Medium risk   ☐ High risk
☐ Refocus   ☐ Move away   ☐ Leave area entirely
I will go: _____

Should I do New-Me Activities?   ☐ Yes   ☐ No
Focus: _____
Feel Good: _____
Distraction: _____
Fun: _____

Should I do Problem Solving?   ☐ Yes   ☐ No   ☐ Yes, when I am calmer
Clear Picture of my problem: _____
Size of the problem: Small   Medium   Large
    Is it a Quick Fix?   ☐ Yes   ☐ No
Check all options:
    Option: _____ 👍 👎
    Option: _____ 👍 👎
    Option: _____ 👍 👎
Plan A: _____
Plan B: _____
Plan C: _____

Should I use Expressing Myself?   ☐ Yes   ☐ No   ☐ Yes, when I am calmer
What do I need to share? _____
Who do I need to share with? _____
How will I share it? _____

(continued)

| **LEARNING SKILLS, USING SKILLS IN MY LIFE** | **WORKSHEET 1**
(page 3 of 3) |

Should I use Getting It Right? ☐ Yes ☐ No ☐ Yes, when I am calmer

Right Mind: _____

Right Person: _____

Right Time and Place: _____

Right Tone: _____

Right Words—Sugar: _____

    Explain: _____

    Ask: _____

    Listen: _____

    Seal a Deal: _____

Should I use Relationship Care? ☐ Yes ☐ No ☐ Yes, when I am calmer

Relationship Care with myself: _____

Relationship Care with others: _____

Should I have a Two-Way-Street relationship by listening and talking? ☐ Yes ☐ No

Should I Find Middle Ground? ☐ Yes ☐ No

Should I do the Steps of Responsibility? ☐ Yes ☐ No

Thumbs-Up Thinking: _____

★ What is my goal? _____

Do I have a Skills Plan? ☐ Yes ☐ No

What will my On-Track Action be? _____

How will I cheer myself on? _____

| LEARNING SKILLS, USING SKILLS IN MY LIFE | **WORKSHEET 2** (page 1 of 2) |

Using My Skills
(when at a Level 4 or 5 feeling)

Name: _____   Date: _____

1. Clear Picture

- Breathe ☐ Yes ☐ No
- Surroundings: _____
- Body Check: _____
- Feeling: _____ Rating: 0–1–2–3–4–5
- Thought: _____
- Urge: _____

2. On-Track Thinking

Check It ☐ 👍 Helpful urge ☐ 👎 Not helpful urge

Turn It 👍 thinking: _____

Cheerleading: _____
_____

Make a Skills Plan: My level of feeling RIGHT NOW: _____

How many skills do I need? _____

What Category of Skills can I use?

    All-the-Time skills 0–5 feeling: ☐ Yes ☐ No

    Calm-Only skills 0–3 feeling: ☐ Yes ☐ No

(continued)

From *The Emotion Regulation Skills System Workbook, Second Edition.* Copyright © 2026 Julie F. Brown. Published by The Guilford Press. Permission to photocopy this material or download it from the epdf is granted to purchasers of this book for personal use; see copyright page for details.

LEARNING SKILLS, USING SKILLS IN MY LIFE

WORKSHEET 2
(page 2 of 2)

Should I use a Safety Plan? Is there any risk? ☐ Yes ☐ No

☐ Thinking   ☐ Talking   ☐ Written
☐ Low risk   ☐ Medium risk   ☐ High risk
☐ Refocus   ☐ Move away   ☐ Leave area entirely
I will go: _____

Should I do New-Me Activities? ☐ Yes ☐ No

Focus: _____
Feel Good: _____
Distraction: _____
Fun: _____

Skills Plan I will use:

Is that enough? ☐ Yes ☐ No

3. On-Track Action: _____

LEARNING SKILLS, USING SKILLS IN MY LIFE

SKILLS CERTIFICATE

Skills Learner: _____

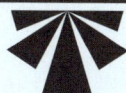

Cycle #: _____   Date: _____

Group Leader: _____

Reaching Goals

The worked examples and worksheets in this section are designed to help you use skills in your life to reach your goals. As you learn skills, you can use these worked examples and worksheets to:

- Create Skills Plans that help you use skills in your life.
- Reflect on how the Skills Plans worked to reach your goals.
- Look back on events to get a Clear Picture about when you were on-track to your goals and off-track from your goals.
- Look forward and think about how you can improve your Skills Plans in the future to help you deal with challenging situations, manage your feelings, and reach your goals.

It might be helpful to work with a skills instructor or therapist to complete these worksheets. Having a partner to reflect with can help us better understand ourselves, our situations, and how to apply skills in our lives.

REACHING GOALS	WORKED EXAMPLE 1

My Skills Plan

Name: _____   Date: _____

Directions: Write down one of your goals and a target you are working on. Create a plan that will help you be on-track to your target and goal. Mark the boxes of skills that will be part of My Plan. Describe how you will use your skills to reach the target in the bottom section of the worksheet.

My Goal _I want to live in an apartment._

My Target _No yelling and hitting this week._
(What I will work on to help me reach My Goal)

My Plan (Skills I will use to reach My Goal)

All-the-Time Skills 0–5 Feelings
- ☒ Clear Picture
- ☒ On-Track Thinking
- ☒ On-Track Actions
- ☒ Safety Plan
- ☒ New-Me Activities

Calm-Only Skills 0–3 Feelings
- ☐ Problem Solving
- ☐ Expressing Myself
- ☐ Getting It Right
- ☐ Relationship Care

My Plan _I will get a Clear Picture every day._
I will think about my goal to get an apartment.
I will do On-Track Thinking. I will Turn off-track thinking—fast!
I will take lots of On-Track Actions all day.
If I get mad at anyone, I will do my Safety Plan and Move Away.
I will do lots of New-Me Activities every day.

From *The Emotion Regulation Skills System Workbook, Second Edition.* Copyright © 2026 Julie F. Brown. Published by The Guilford Press. Permission to photocopy this material or download it from the epdf is granted to purchasers of this book for personal use; see copyright page for details.

REACHING GOALS — WORKSHEET 1

My Skills Plan

Name: _____ Date: _____

Directions: Write down one of your goals and a target you are working on. Create a plan that will help you be on-track to your target and goal. Mark the boxes of skills that will be part of My Plan. Describe how you will use your skills to reach the target in the bottom section of the worksheet.

My Goal _____

My Target _____
(What I will work on to help me reach My Goal)

My Plan (Skills I will use to reach My Goal)

All-the-Time Skills 0–5 Feelings
- ☐ Clear Picture
- ☐ On-Track Thinking
- ☐ On-Track Actions
- ☐ Safety Plan
- ☐ New-Me Activities

Calm-Only Skills 0–3 Feelings
- ☐ Problem Solving
- ☐ Expressing Myself
- ☐ Getting It Right
- ☐ Relationship Care

My Plan _____

_____

_____

_____

_____

From *The Emotion Regulation Skills System Workbook, Second Edition*. Copyright © 2026 Julie F. Brown. Published by The Guilford Press. Permission to photocopy this material or download it from the epdf is granted to purchasers of this book for personal use; see copyright page for details.

| REACHING GOALS | WORKED EXAMPLE 2 |

My Diary Card

Name: _____   Date: _____

Directions: It can be helpful to track our progress on targets during the week. Write down the target you are working on at the top. Each evening write down the date and check whether you had On-Track Actions, Off-Track Urges, or Off-Track Actions related to the target. Describe the urges and/or actions below the check boxes. Use the back if you need more space to write.

🎯 Target: _____

Monday—Date: __2/10__   ☒ On-Track Actions   ☐ Off-Track Urges   ☐ Off-Track Actions
Describe: _I did my laundry. I worked on my puzzle._

Tuesday—Date: __2/11__   ☒ On-Track Actions   ☒ Off-Track Urges   ☐ Off-Track Actions
Describe: _I wanted to yell at my housemate. He was super loud. I used my headphones and stayed in my room._

Wednesday—Date: __2/12__   ☒ On-Track Actions   ☐ Off-Track Urges   ☐ Off-Track Actions
Describe: _I did my chores. I called my sister. I did my puzzle._

Thursday—Date: __2/13__   ☒ On-Track Actions   ☐ Off-Track Urges   ☐ Off-Track Actions
Describe: _I went on the computer. I went grocery shopping._

Friday—Date: __2/14__   ☐ On-Track Actions   ☐ Off-Track Urges   ☒ Off-Track Actions
Describe: _Staff was rude. He is bossy. I told him off. I punched the wall._

Saturday—Date: __2/15__   ☒ On-Track Actions   ☐ Off-Track Urges   ☐ Off-Track Actions
Describe: _Went to the doctor for my hand. Took a nap._

Sunday—Date: __2/16__   ☒ On-Track Actions   ☐ Off-Track Urges   ☐ Off-Track Actions
Describe: _Saw my sister at the park. Did my chores after._

From *The Emotion Regulation Skills System Workbook, Second Edition.* Copyright © 2026 Julie F. Brown. Published by The Guilford Press. Permission to photocopy this material or download it from the epdf is granted to purchasers of this book for personal use; see copyright page for details.

| REACHING GOALS | WORKSHEET 2 |

My Diary Card

Name: _____   Date: _____

Directions: It can be helpful to track our progress on targets during the week. Write down the target you are working on at the top. Each evening write down the date and check whether you had On-Track Actions, Off-Track Urges, or Off-Track Actions related to the target. Describe the urges and/or actions below the check boxes. Use the back if you need more space to write.

🎯 Target: _____

| Monday—Date: _____   ☐ On-Track Actions   ☐ Off-Track Urges   ☐ Off-Track Actions |
| Describe: _____ |

| Tuesday—Date: _____   ☐ On-Track Actions   ☐ Off-Track Urges   ☐ Off-Track Actions |
| Describe: _____ |

| Wednesday—Date: _____   ☐ On-Track Actions   ☐ Off-Track Urges   ☐ Off-Track Actions |
| Describe: _____ |

| Thursday—Date: _____   ☐ On-Track Actions   ☐ Off-Track Urges   ☐ Off-Track Actions |
| Describe: _____ |

| Friday—Date: _____   ☐ On-Track Actions   ☐ Off-Track Urges   ☐ Off-Track Actions |
| Describe: _____ |

| Saturday—Date: _____   ☐ On-Track Actions   ☐ Off-Track Urges   ☐ Off-Track Actions |
| Describe: _____ |

| Sunday—Date: _____   ☐ On-Track Actions   ☐ Off-Track Urges   ☐ Off-Track Actions |
| Describe: _____ |

From *The Emotion Regulation Skills System Workbook, Second Edition*. Copyright © 2026 Julie F. Brown. Published by The Guilford Press. Permission to photocopy this material or download it from the epdf is granted to purchasers of this book for personal use; see copyright page for details.

| REACHING GOALS | WORKED EXAMPLE 3 |

My Progress

Name: _____ Date: _____

Directions: Thinking about how you are moving toward your targets each day or each week can help you make progress toward your goals. Write down any target that you are working on. Use a separate My Progress worksheet for each target. List On-Track Actions you have taken that helped you move toward the target. Then write down any Off-Track Urges and Off-Track Actions you have had. At the bottom, write down any targets you want to continue to work on. It may help you reach your goal if you make a new My Skills Plan for each new target you want to work on.

My Goal _____ I want to have my own apartment. _____

My Target _____ No yelling and hitting this week. _____
(What I will work on to help me reach My Goal)

My Progress: On-Track Actions   **Day:**

I put my headphones on when my housemate was loud.   Tuesday

I did my puzzle and stayed in my room.   Tuesday

I took my medications all week.   All

Off-Track Urges   **Day:**

I wanted to yell at my housemate.   Tuesday

I wanted to skip my medications.   Friday

Off-Track Actions   **Day:**

My staff was bossing me around and being rude.   Friday

I told him off and punched a wall.   Friday

Moving Ahead:

Would it help to do a Back-Track and Re-Track?   ☒ Yes   ☐ No

What situation will you Back-Track and Re-Track?   Friday—when I punched a wall.

Would it help to make a new Skills Plan?   ☒ Yes   ☐ No

From *The Emotion Regulation Skills System Workbook, Second Edition*. Copyright © 2026 Julie F. Brown. Published by The Guilford Press. Permission to photocopy this material or download it from the epdf is granted to purchasers of this book for personal use; see copyright page for details.

REACHING GOALS	WORKSHEET 3

My Progress

Name: _____   Date: _____

Directions: Thinking about how you are moving toward your targets each day or each week can help you make progress toward your goals. Write down any target that you are working on. Use a separate My Progress worksheet for each target. List On-Track Actions you have taken that helped you move toward the target. Then write down any Off-Track Urges and Off-Track Actions you have had. At the bottom, write down any targets you want to continue to work on. It may help you reach your goal if you make a new My Skills Plan for each new target you want to work on.

My Goal _____

My Target _____
(What I will work on to help me reach My Goal)

My Progress: On-Track Actions   Day:
_____
_____

Off-Track Urges   Day:
_____

Off-Track Actions   Day:
_____
_____

Moving Ahead:

Would it help to do a Back-Track and Re-Track?   ☐ Yes   ☐ No
What situation will you Back-Track and Re-Track? _____
Would it help to make a new Skills Plan?   ☐ Yes   ☐ No

From *The Emotion Regulation Skills System Workbook, Second Edition*. Copyright © 2026 Julie F. Brown. Published by The Guilford Press. Permission to photocopy this material or download it from the epdf is granted to purchasers of this book for personal use; see copyright page for details.

REACHING GOALS — WORKED EXAMPLE 4

Back-Track

Name: _____ Date: _____ Situation: Punched a wall

Directions: Think of a situation that you would like to Back-Track. For each level of feeling you experienced, fill in the Clear Picture Do's and actions you took.

5
- Breath: Fast
- Surroundings: My bedroom
- Body Check: Fist tight
- Feeling: Mad 5
- Thought: I'm stuck here
- Urge: Punch staff
- ACTION → Punched the wall.

4
- Breath: Fast
- Surroundings: Staff banged on my door
- Body Check: Tight neck
- Feeling: Mad 4
- Thought: I hate him
- Urge: Yell at him
- ACTION → Told staff not to tell me what to do.

3
- Breath: Shallow
- Surroundings: Staff told me to come do dishes
- Body Check: Heart beating fast
- Feeling: Upset 3
- Thought: I don't like his attitude
- Urge: Tell him to shut up
- ACTION → I didn't answer the staff.

2
- Breath: Kinda fast
- Surroundings: Staff told me to come do dishes
- Body Check: Tensing up
- Feeling: Frustrated 2
- Thought: He is annoying
- Urge: Tell him to stop
- ACTION → Put my headphones on and listen to music.

1
- Breath: Slow
- Surroundings: My room
- Body Check: Tired
- Feeling: Bored 1
- Thought: I want to chill out
- Urge: Take a nap
- ACTION → Lay on my bed.

From *The Emotion Regulation Skills System Workbook, Second Edition.* Copyright © 2026 Julie F. Brown. Published by The Guilford Press. Permission to photocopy this material or download it from the epdf is granted to purchasers of this book for personal use; see copyright page for details.

REACHING GOALS WORKSHEET 4

Back-Track

Name: _____ Date: _____ Situation: _____

Directions: Think of a situation that you would like to Back-Track. For each level of feeling you experienced, fill in the Clear Picture Do's and actions you took.

5
- Breath:
- Surroundings:
- Body Check:
- Feeling:
- Thought:
- Urge:
- ACTION: _____

4
- Breath:
- Surroundings:
- Body Check:
- Feeling:
- Thought:
- Urge:
- ACTION: _____

3
- Breath:
- Surroundings:
- Body Check:
- Feeling:
- Thought:
- Urge:
- ACTION: _____

2
- Breath:
- Surroundings:
- Body Check:
- Feeling:
- Thought:
- Urge:
- ACTION: _____

1
- Breath:
- Surroundings:
- Body Check:
- Feeling:
- Thought:
- Urge:
- ACTION: _____

From *The Emotion Regulation Skills System Workbook, Second Edition*. Copyright © 2026 Julie F. Brown. Published by The Guilford Press. Permission to photocopy this material or download it from the epdf is granted to purchasers of this book for personal use; see copyright page for details.

| REACHING GOALS | WORKED EXAMPLE 5 |

Re-Track

Name: _____ Date: _____ Situation: <u>Not punching a wall</u>

Directions: After doing a Back-Track, circle whether each ACTION was on-track or off-track from your goal. If on-track, write down any additional skills you could have used. If off-track, Turn It and make a new Skills Plan.

5 Check It:
Circle: On-Track / Off-Track
- Turn It: <u>Punching walls makes things worse.</u>
- Cheerleading: <u>I can get back on-track!</u>
- Skills Plan: <u>I will lie down on my bed. I will stay in my room and do my relaxation exercises.</u>
- Circle: (skill icons)

4 Check It:
Circle: On-Track / Off-Track
- Turn It: <u>I'm working on not yelling at people.</u>
- Cheerleading: <u>I want to move out of here!</u>
- Skills Plan: <u>I will focus on doing the dishes. I will not yell at staff. When I'm done, I'll do my puzzle.</u>
- Circle: (skill icons)

3 Check It:
Circle: On-Track / Off-Track
- Turn It: <u>If I do my chore now it will be done.</u>
- Cheerleading: <u>Doing dishes is a New-Me Activity!</u>
- Skills Plan: <u>I will do my chore today and talk to the manager tomorrow about the staff being rude.</u>
- Circle: (skill icons)

2 Check It:
Circle: On-Track / Off-Track
- Turn It: <u>I have to work with staff and not yell.</u>
- Cheerleading: <u>I want to stay on-track to my goals.</u>
- Skills Plan: <u>Go see what he wants. Take a few belly breaths. Listen and take On-Track Actions.</u>
- Circle: (skill icons)

1 Check It:
Circle: On-Track / Off-Track
- Turn It:
- Cheerleading: <u>I have been on-track today!</u>
- Skills Plan: <u>I will chill out in my room and do my puzzle. I will wear headphones if it gets loud.</u>
- Circle: (skill icons)

From *The Emotion Regulation Skills System Workbook, Second Edition*. Copyright © 2026 Julie F. Brown. Published by The Guilford Press. Permission to photocopy this material or download it from the epdf is granted to purchasers of this book for personal use; see copyright page for details.

| REACHING GOALS | WORKSHEET 5 |

Re-Track

Name: _____ Date: _____ Situation: _____

Directions: After doing a Back-Track, circle whether each ACTION was on-track or off-track from your goal. If on-track, write down any additional skills you could have used. If off-track, Turn It and make a new Skills Plan.

5 Check It:
Circle:
On-Track 👍
Off-Track 👎

Turn It: _____
Cheerleading: _____
Skills Plan: _____
Circle: 🖥 🧠 🚂 🛡 ☕ 📻 ⛄ 📦 🚢

4 Check It:
Circle:
On-Track 👍
Off-Track 👎

Turn It: _____
Cheerleading: _____
Skills Plan: _____
Circle: 🖥 🧠 🚂 🛡 ☕ 📻 ⛄ 📦 🚢

3 Check It:
Circle:
On-Track 👍
Off-Track 👎

Turn It: _____
Cheerleading: _____
Skills Plan: _____
Circle: 🖥 🧠 🚂 🛡 ☕ 📻 ⛄ 📦 🚢

2 Check It:
Circle:
On-Track 👍
Off-Track 👎

Turn It: _____
Cheerleading: _____
Skills Plan: _____
Circle: 🖥 🧠 🚂 🛡 ☕ 📻 ⛄ 📦 🚢

1 Check It:
Circle:
On-Track 👍
Off-Track 👎

Turn It: _____
Cheerleading: _____
Skills Plan: _____
Circle: 🖥 🧠 🚂 🛡 ☕ 📻 ⛄ 📦 🚢

From *The Emotion Regulation Skills System Workbook, Second Edition*. Copyright © 2026 Julie F. Brown. Published by The Guilford Press. Permission to photocopy this material or download it from the epdf is granted to purchasers of this book for personal use; see copyright page for details.

Index

Accept the Situation. *See also* On-Track Action; Situations
  Accept the Situation and Turn the Page worksheet, 120–121
  Accepting the Situation handout, 118
  Examples of On-Track Actions worksheet, 122–123
  Five Types of On-Track Actions handout, 105
  overview, 103
  Problem Solving, 159
  Relationship Care, 198
Accept the Situation and Turn the Page worksheet, 120–121
Accepting the Situation handout, 118
Action Urges by Feelings Level worksheet, 76–77
All-the-Time Skills. *See also* Clear Picture; New-Me Activities; On-Track Action; On-Track Thinking; Safety Plan; Skills List
  Categories of Skills handout, 36
  Feelings Ratings and Categories of Skills worksheet, 40
  How I Use the Skills System handout, 31
  How Our Skills Help Us handout, 24
  On-Track Thinking and, 85
  overview, 51
  Recipe for Skills handout, 41
  Review Questions, 47
  Select the Category of Skills by Feeling Level worksheet, 38–39
  Skills Plan Map, 219
  Using My Skills worksheets, 220–224
Automatic thoughts. *See* Notice My Thoughts

Back-Track, 235–236
Back-Track worksheet, 235–236
Balance
  Balancing in My Life worksheet, 115
  Balancing My Life worksheet, 116–117
  Balancing On-Track Relationships handout, 203
  Balancing On-Track Relationships: One- and Two-Way Streets handout, 204

Building, Balancing, and Changing Relationships handout, 199
Expressing Myself, 173
My On-Track Action Plan worksheet, 113–114
On-Track Action Plans handout, 112
Relationship Care, 197
Balancing in My Life worksheet, 115
Balancing My Life worksheet, 116–117
Balancing On-Track Relationships handout, 203
Balancing On-Track Relationships: One- and Two-Way Streets handout, 204
Balancing On-Track Relationships worksheet, 205
Body Check. *See also* Clear Picture
  Accept the Situation and Turn the Page worksheet, 120–121
  Body Check as a Focus New-Me Activity (exercise 1), 148
  Body Check: Sensations by Feelings Level worksheet, 61–62
  Body Check worksheet, 59–60
  Clear Picture Do's handout, 52
  Getting a Clear Picture worksheet, 53–54
  overview, 51
Body Check as a Focus New-Me Activity (exercise 1), 148
Body Check: Sensations by Feelings Level worksheet, 61–62
Body Check worksheet, 59–60
Body language, 173, 174, 178. *See also* Expressing Myself
Breath, 92–93, 120–121, 235–236. *See also* Notice My Breath
Build On-Track Relationships, 197, 199, 200, 201, 202. *See also* Relationship Care
Build Your Recipe for Skills worksheet, 44
Building, Balancing, and Changing Relationships handout, 199
Building a Safety Plan worksheet, 135
Building On-Track Relationships: Different Types of Relationships handout, 202

Building On-Track Relationships handout, 200
Building On-Track Relationships worksheet, 201

Calm-Only Skills. *See also* Expressing Myself; Getting It Right; Problem Solving; Relationship Care; Skills List
  Categories of Skills handout, 36
  Feelings Ratings and Categories of Skills worksheet, 40
  How I Use the Skills System handout, 31
  How Our Skills Help Us handout, 24
  On-Track Thinking and, 85
  Recipe for Skills handout, 41
  Review Questions, 47
  Select the Category of Skills by Feeling Level worksheet, 38–39
  Skills Plan Map, 219
  Using My Skills worksheets, 220–224
Categories of Skills. *See also* System Tools
  Categories of Skills handout, 36
  How I Use the Skills System handout, 31
  Name the Skills and Categories of Skills worksheet, 37
  overview, 19, 31
  Review Questions, 47
  Select the Category of Skills by Feeling Level worksheet, 38–39
  Skills Plan, 85
  Week 2 Practice Activity worksheet, 45–46
Categories of Skills handout, 36
Certificate, Skills, 225
Changing Off-Track Relationships handouts, 206, 212
Check All Options, 159, 162, 165–166, 169–170. *See also* Problem Solving
Check All Options worksheet, 165–166
Check It. *See also* On-Track Thinking
  Check It worksheet, 89
  On-Track Action, 103
  On-Track Thinking: Create a Skills Plan worksheet, 92–93

Index

Check It (*cont.*)
On-Track Thinking Through a Situation worksheet, 87–88
overview, 85
Turn It worksheet, 90–91
Check It worksheet, 89
Check My Surroundings. *See also* Clear Picture
Accept the Situation and Turn the Page worksheet, 120–121
Clear Picture Do's handout, 52
Getting a Clear Picture worksheet, 53–54
Notice Surroundings handout, 56
Notice Surroundings worksheet, 57–58
On-Track Thinking: Create a Skills Plan worksheet, 92–93
overview, 51
Cheerleading. *See also* On-Track Thinking
Cheerleading: Blast It worksheet, 94–95
On-Track Action, 103
On-Track Thinking: Create a Skills Plan worksheet, 92–93
On-Track Thinking Through a Situation worksheet, 87–88
On-Track Thinking to Meet My Goals handout, 86
overview, 85
Turn It worksheet, 90–91
Cheerleading: Blast It worksheet, 94–95
Clear Picture. *See also* All-the-Time Skills; Body Check; Check My Surroundings; Label and Rate My Feelings; Learning Skills activities; Notice My Breath; Notice My Thoughts; Notice My Urges
Accept the Situation and Turn the Page worksheet, 120–121
Action Urges by Feelings Level worksheet, 76–77
Body Check: Sensations by Feelings Level worksheet, 61–62
Body Check worksheet, 59–60
Categories of Skills handout, 36
Changing Off-Track Relationships handout, 206
Clear Picture Do's handout, 52
Clear Picture of the Problem worksheet, 163–164
Expressing Myself, 173, 180
Expressing Myself Self-Check worksheet, 180
Feelings and Their Action Urges worksheet, 74–75
Getting a Clear Picture worksheet, 53–54
How Our Skills Help Us handout, 24
Label and Rate Feelings: How Feelings Affect Me handout, 64
Label and Rate Feelings in Specific Situations worksheet, 65–66

Label and Rate Feelings: List of Feelings and Emotions handout, 63
Nine Core Skills handout, 23
Notice My Breath worksheet, 55
Notice Surroundings handout, 56
Notice Surroundings worksheet, 57–58
Noticing My Reactions worksheet, 80–81
Noticing My Thoughts handout, 67
Noticing Thoughts at Different Feelings Levels worksheet, 70–71
On-Track Action, 103
On-Track Action: Switching Tracks worksheet, 110–111
On-Track Thinking and, 85
overview, 19, 24, 51
Reaching Goals activities, 227
Relationship Care, 197, 198
Relationship Check worksheet, 207–208
Right Person handout, 189
Right Tone handout, 191
Right Words—SEALS handout, 192
Safety Plan, 127
Situations that Lead to Noticing Thoughts worksheet, 68–69
Situations that Lead to Noticing Urges worksheet, 78–79
Skills Chain, 85
Skills Plan Map, 219
Solo and Partnership New-Me Activities handout, 145
Switch Tracks to On-Track Action handout, 109
Take a Step toward My Goal in Wise Mind handout, 106
Thoughts and Feelings Lead to Urges worksheet, 72–73
Turn the Page handout, 119
Using My Skills worksheets, 220–224
Written Safety Plan worksheet, 137–138
Clear Picture Do's, 52, 235–236. *See also* Clear Picture
Clear Picture Do's handout, 52
Clear Picture of the Problem, 159, 160–161, 162, 163–164, 169–170. *See also* Clear Picture; Problem Solving
Clear Picture of the Problem worksheet, 163–164
Clear Picture of the Risk, 127
Communication, 173, 178. *See also* Expressing Myself
Core Self, 197

Detailed Safety Plan worksheet, 139–140
Diary cards, 231–232
Distraction Activities, 143, 144, 151, 152, 155–156. *See also* New-Me Activities
Distraction New-Me Activities handout, 151

Ending relationships, 209. *See also* Relationship Care
Environment. *See* Check My Surroundings
Examples of High, Medium, and Low Risks worksheet, 132–133
Examples of Inside and Outside Risks worksheet, 129–130
Examples of On-Track Actions worksheet, 122–123
Exploring My Goals worksheet, 13–14
Exploring Targets to Reach My Goal worksheet, 15–16
Expressing Myself. *See also* Calm-Only Skills; In My Heart; Learning Skills activities; On My Mind
Categories of Skills handout, 36
Examples of On-Track Actions worksheet, 122–123
Expressing Myself Plan worksheet, 181–182
Expressing Myself Self-Check worksheet, 180
Expressing What's On My Mind and In My Heart worksheet, 175–176
Finding Middle Ground handout, 209
How Do I Use Expressing Myself? handout, 178
How Our Skills Help Us handout, 24
Nine Core Skills handout, 23
123 Wise Mind worksheet, 124
overview, 19, 24, 173
Relationship Care, 198
Skills Chain, 85
Skills Plan, 85, 219
Summary Sheet, 173
Take a Step toward My Goal in Wise Mind handout, 106
Using My Skills worksheets, 220–224
What Is Expressing Myself handout, 174
When Do I Use Expressing Myself? handout, 179
Why Do I Express Myself? handout, 177
Expressing Myself Plan worksheet, 181–182
Expressing Myself Self-Check worksheet, 180
Expressing What's On My Mind and In My Heart worksheet, 175–176

Fantasies, 129–130
Feel Good Activities, 143, 144, 149, 150, 155–156. *See also* New-Me Activities
Feel Good New-Me Activities handout, 149
Feelings. *See also* Feelings Rating Scale; Label and Rate My Feelings; Level of feelings
Action Urges by Feelings Level worksheet, 76–77
Back-Track worksheet, 235–236
Body Check: Sensations by Feelings Level worksheet, 61–62

Index

Changing Off-Track Relationships handout, 212
Examples of Inside and Outside Risks worksheet, 129–130
Expressing Myself, 173, 180
Expressing Myself Self-Check worksheet, 180
Feelings and Their Action Urges worksheet, 74–75
Feelings Rating Scale with Descriptions handout, 33
Feelings Rating Scale with Pictures handout, 32
Feelings Rating Scale worksheet, 34–35
Feelings Ratings and Categories of Skills worksheet, 40
Getting to Know My Feelings worksheet, 7–8
How I Use the Skills System handout, 31
Label and Rate Feelings: How Feelings Affect Me handout, 64
Label and Rate Feelings in Specific Situations worksheet, 65–66
Label and Rate Feelings: List of Feelings and Emotions handout, 63
New-Me Activities, 143
Noticing My Reactions worksheet, 80–81
Noticing Thoughts at Different Feelings Levels worksheet, 70–71
On-Track Thinking: Create a Skills Plan worksheet, 92–93
Recipe for Skills handout, 41
Select the Category of Skills by Feeling Level worksheet, 38–39
Thoughts and Feelings Lead to Urges worksheet, 72–73
When Do I Use Expressing Myself? handout, 179
Why Do I Express Myself? handout, 177
Feelings and Their Action Urges worksheet, 74–75
Feelings Rating Scale. *See also* Feelings; System Tools
  Feelings Rating Scale with Descriptions handout, 33
  Feelings Rating Scale with Pictures handout, 32
  Feelings Rating Scale worksheet, 34–35
  How I Use the Skills System handout, 31
  overview, 19, 31
  Review Questions, 47
  Week 2 Practice Activity worksheet, 45–46
Feelings Rating Scale with Descriptions handout, 33
Feelings Rating Scale with Pictures handout, 32
Feelings Rating Scale worksheet, 34–35

Feelings Ratings and Categories of Skills worksheet, 40
Finding Middle Ground, 173, 198, 199, 209, 210–211. *See also* Relationship Care
Finding Middle Ground handout, 209
Finding Middle Ground Plan worksheet, 210–211
Five Types of On-Track Actions handout, 105
Focus Activities. *See also* New-Me Activities
  Body Check as a Focus New-Me Activity (exercise 1), 148
  Focus New-Me Activities handout, 146
  My Focus New-Me Activities worksheet, 147
  overview, 143
  Solo New-Me Activities and Self-Care worksheet, 155–156
  Types of New-Me Activities handout, 144
Focus New-Me Activities handout, 146
Focus on a New-Me Activity. *See also* New-Me Activities; Safety Plan
  Building a Safety Plan worksheet, 136
  Detailed Safety Plan worksheet, 139–140
  overview, 127, 143
  Three Ways to Handle Risk handout, 135
  Written Safety Plan worksheet, 137–138
Fun Activities, 143, 144, 153, 154, 155–156. *See also* New-Me Activities
Fun New-Me Activities handout, 153

Getting a Clear Picture of the Risk: Three Levels of Risk handout, 131
Getting a Clear Picture worksheet, 53–54
Getting It Right. *See also* Calm-Only Skills; Learning Skills activities; Right Mind; Right Person; Right Time and Place; Right Tone; Right Words: SEALS
  Categories of Skills handout, 36
  Examples of On-Track Actions worksheet, 122–123
  Expressing Myself, 173, 180
  Expressing Myself Self-Check worksheet, 180
  Finding Middle Ground handout, 209
  Getting It Right Plan worksheet, 193–194
  Getting What I Want! handout, 186
  How Our Skills Help Us handout, 24
  Nine Core Skills handout, 23
  123 Wise Mind worksheet, 124
  On-Track Action, 103
  overview, 19, 24, 185
  Relationship Care, 198
  Right Mind handout, 187

Right Mind Self-Check worksheet, 188
Right Person handout, 189
Right Time and Place handout, 190
Right Tone handout, 191
Right Words—SEALS handout, 192
Skills Chain, 85
Skills Plan, 85, 219
Summary Sheet, 185
Take a Step toward My Goal in Wise Mind handout, 106
Using My Skills worksheets, 220–224
Why Do I Express Myself? handout, 177
Getting It Right Plan worksheet, 193–194
Getting to Know Me worksheet, 5–6
Getting to Know My Feelings worksheet, 7–8
Getting What I Want! handout, 186
Goals. *See also* Reaching Goals activities; Take a Step toward My Goal
  Check It worksheet, 89
  Clear Picture of the Problem worksheet, 163–164
  exploring, 2, 3
  Exploring My Goals worksheet, 13–14
  Exploring Targets to Reach My Goal worksheet, 15–16
  Five Types of On-Track Actions handout, 105
  My Diary Card worksheet, 231–232
  My Goals worksheet, 11–12
  My New-Me and My Old Me worksheet, 9–10
  My Progress worksheet, 233–234
  My Skills Plan worksheet, 229–230
  On- and Off-Tracks handout, 104
  On-Track Actions and My Goals worksheet, 107–108
  On-Track Thinking to Meet My Goals handout, 86
  Relationship Care, 198
  Take a Step toward My Goal in Wise Mind handout, 106
  Turn It worksheet, 90–91

Handouts, 1, 2. *See also* Worksheets; *individual handouts*
Happiness, 143, 153
High-risk situations. *See also* Risks; Situations
  Building a Safety Plan worksheet, 136
  Detailed Safety Plan worksheet, 139–140
  Examples of High, Medium, and Low Risks worksheet, 132–133
  Getting a Clear Picture of the Risk: Three Levels of Risk handout, 131
  Safety Plan, 127, 136, 137–138, 139–140
  Three Ways to Handle Risk handout, 135
  Written Safety Plan worksheet, 137–138

Index

How Do I Use Expressing Myself? handout, 178
How I Use the Skills System handout, 31
How Our Skills Help Us handout, 24

Impulses. *See* Notice My Urges; Urges
In My Heart, 173, 174, 175–176, 177. *See also* Expressing Myself
Inside and Outside Risks handout, 128
Inside Risks, 127, 128, 129–130, 136. *See also* Risks

Jump in with Both Feet, 103, 109, 110–111, 173. *See also* On-Track Action

Label and Rate Feelings: How Feelings Affect Me handout, 64
Label and Rate Feelings in Specific Situations worksheet, 65–66
Label and Rate Feelings: List of Feelings and Emotions handout, 63
Label and Rate My Feelings. *See also* Clear Picture; Feelings
  Accept the Situation and Turn the Page worksheet, 120–121
  Clear Picture Do's handout, 52
  Getting a Clear Picture worksheet, 53–54
  Label and Rate Feelings: How Feelings Affect Me handout, 64
  Label and Rate Feelings in Specific Situations worksheet, 65–66
  Label and Rate Feelings: List of Feelings and Emotions handout, 63
  overview, 51
Learning Skills activities, 2, 17, 19. *See also* Clear Picture; Expressing Myself; Getting It Right; New-Me Activities; On-Track Action; On-Track Thinking; Problem Solving; Relationship Care; Safety Plan; Skills List; System Tools
Leave the Area, 127, 135, 136, 137–138, 139–140. *See also* Safety Plan
Let Go and Move On, 122–123
Level of feelings. *See also* Feelings; Feelings Rating Scale
  Action Urges by Feelings Level worksheet, 76–77
  Body Check: Sensations by Feelings Level worksheet, 61–62
  Build Your Recipe for Skills worksheet, 44
  Clear Picture, 51
  Expressing Myself, 173, 180
  Expressing Myself Self-Check worksheet, 180
  Feel Good New-Me Activities handout, 149
  Feelings Rating Scale with Descriptions handout, 33
  Feelings Rating Scale with Pictures handout, 32
  Feelings Ratings and Categories of Skills worksheet, 40
  Feelings Ratings Scale worksheet, 34–35
  Getting It Right, 185
  How I Use the Skills System handout, 31
  Noticing Thoughts at Different Feelings Levels worksheet, 70–71
  On-Track Action, 103
  On-Track Thinking: Create a Skills Plan worksheet, 92–93
  Problem Solving, 159, 162
  Recipe for Skills: Choose How Many Skills to Use worksheet, 42–43
  Recipe for Skills handout, 41
  Right Mind handout, 187
  Select the Category of Skills by Feeling Level worksheet, 38–39
  Skills Plan, 85, 219
  When Do I Use Expressing Myself? handout, 179
Low-risk situations. *See also* Risks; Situations
  Building a Safety Plan worksheet, 136
  Detailed Safety Plan worksheet, 139–140
  Examples of High, Medium, and Low Risks worksheet, 132–133
  Getting a Clear Picture of the Risk: Three Levels of Risk handout, 131
  Safety Plan, 127
  Three Ways to Handle Risk handout, 135
  Written Safety Plan worksheet, 137–138

Make Plans A, B, and C worksheet, 167–168
Match the Skill Number and Initial to the Picture worksheet, 26
Medium-risk situations. *See also* Risks; Situations
  Building a Safety Plan worksheet, 136
  Detailed Safety Plan worksheet, 139–140
  Examples of High, Medium, and Low Risks worksheet, 132–133
  Getting a Clear Picture of the Risk: Three Levels of Risk handout, 131
  Safety Plan, 127
  Three Ways to Handle Risk handout, 135
  Written Safety Plan worksheet, 137–138
Move Away, 127, 136, 137–138, 139–140. *See also* Safety Plan
My Diary Card worksheet, 231–232
My Distraction New-Me Activities worksheet, 152
My Feel Good New-Me Activities worksheet, 150
My Focus New-Me Activities worksheet, 147
My Fun New-Me Activities worksheet, 154
My Goals worksheet, 11–12
My New-Me and My Old Me worksheet, 9–10
My On-Track Action Plan worksheet, 113–114
My Progress worksheet, 233–234
My Skills Plan worksheet, 229–230

Name the Skill by Number worksheet, 27
Name the Skill by Picture worksheet, 25
Name the Skills and Categories of Skills worksheet, 37
New-Me Activities. *See also* All-the-Time Skills; Distraction Activities; Feel Good Activities; Focus Activities; Focus on a New-Me Activity; Fun Activities; Learning Skills activities; Partnership New-Me Activities; Solo New-Me Activities
  Body Check as a Focus New-Me Activity (exercise 1), 148
  Building a Safety Plan worksheet, 136
  Categories of Skills handout, 36
  Changing Off-Track Relationships handout, 206
  Detailed Safety Plan worksheet, 139–140
  Distraction New-Me Activities handout, 151
  Examples of On-Track Actions worksheet, 122–123
  Expressing Myself, 173
  Feel Good New-Me Activities handout, 149
  Focus New-Me Activities handout, 146
  Fun New-Me Activities handout, 153
  How Our Skills Help Us handout, 24
  My Distraction New-Me Activities worksheet, 152
  My Feel Good New-Me Activities worksheet, 150
  My Focus New-Me Activities worksheet, 147
  My Fun New-Me Activities worksheet, 154
  Nine Core Skills handout, 23
  123 Wise Mind worksheet, 124
  On-Track Action: Switching Tracks worksheet, 110–111
  overview, 19, 24, 143
  Skills Chain, 85
  Skills Plan, 85, 219
  Solo and Partnership New-Me Activities handout, 145
  Solo New-Me Activities and Self-Care worksheet, 155–156
  Summary Sheet, 143
  Take a Step toward My Goal in Wise Mind handout, 106

Index

Three Ways to Handle Risk handout, 135
Turn the Page handout, 119
Types of New-Me Activities handout, 144
Using My Skills worksheets, 220–224
What Is Expressing Myself handout, 174
When Do I Use Expressing Myself? handout, 179
Written Safety Plan worksheet, 137–138
Nine Core Skills handout, 23
Notice My Breath, 51, 52, 53–54, 55. *See also* Breath; Clear Picture
Notice My Breath worksheet, 55
Notice My Surroundings. *See* Check My Surroundings
Notice My Thoughts. *See also* Clear Picture; Thoughts
  Clear Picture Do's handout, 52
  Getting a Clear Picture worksheet, 53–54
  Noticing My Thoughts handout, 67
  Noticing Thoughts at Different Feelings Levels worksheet, 70–71
  On-Track Thinking: Create a Skills Plan worksheet, 92–93
  overview, 51
  Situations that Lead to Noticing Thoughts worksheet, 68–69
  Thoughts and Feelings Lead to Urges worksheet, 72–73
Notice My Urges. *See also* Clear Picture; Urges
  Action Urges by Feelings Level worksheet, 76–77
  Clear Picture Do's handout, 52
  Feelings and Their Action Urges worksheet, 74–75
  Getting a Clear Picture worksheet, 53–54
  Noticing My Reactions worksheet, 80–81
  On-Track Thinking: Create a Skills Plan worksheet, 92–93
  overview, 51
  Situations that Lead to Noticing Urges worksheet, 78–79
  Thoughts and Feelings Lead to Urges worksheet, 72–73
Notice Surroundings handout, 56
Notice Surroundings worksheet, 57–58
Noticing My Reactions worksheet, 80–81
Noticing My Thoughts handout, 67
Noticing Thoughts at Different Feelings Levels worksheet, 70–71

Off-Track Actions, 9–10, 104, 151, 231–232, 233–234, 237–238. *See also* On-Track Action
Off-Track Relationships, 198, 206. *See also* Relationship Care
Off-Track Thoughts, 51, 90–91, 92–93, 94–95. *See also* Notice My Thoughts; On-Track Thinking; Thoughts
Off-Track Urges, 109, 110–111, 231–232, 233–234. *See also* Urges
On- and Off-Tracks handout, 104
On My Mind, 173, 174, 175–176, 177. *See also* Expressing Myself
123 Wise Mind, 85, 104, 124. *See also* Wise Mind
123 Wise Mind worksheet, 124
One-Way-Street Relationship, 198, 199, 204, 205. *See also* Relationship Care
On-Track Action. *See also* Accept the Situation; All-the-Time Skills; Jump in with Both Feet; Learning Skills activities; On-Track Action Plans; Opposite Action; Switch Tracks; Take a Step toward My Goal; Turn the Page
  Accept the Situation and Turn the Page worksheet, 120–121
  Accepting the Situation handout, 118
  Balancing in My Life worksheet, 115
  Balancing My Life worksheet, 116–117
  Categories of Skills handout, 36
  Changing Off-Track Relationships handout, 206
  Clear Picture and, 51
  Examples of On-Track Actions worksheet, 122–123
  Expressing Myself, 173, 180
  Expressing Myself Self-Check worksheet, 180
  Five Types of On-Track Actions handout, 105
  Fun New-Me Activities handout, 153
  How Our Skills Help Us handout, 24
  My Diary Card worksheet, 231–232
  My On-Track Action Plan worksheet, 113–114
  My Progress worksheet, 233–234
  Nine Core Skills handout, 23
  On- and Off-Tracks handout, 104
  123 Wise Mind worksheet, 124
  On-Track Action Plans handout, 112
  On-Track Action: Switching Tracks worksheet, 110–111
  On-Track Actions and My Goals worksheet, 107–108
  On-Track Thinking Through a Situation worksheet, 87–88
  On-Track Thinking to Meet My Goals handout, 86
  overview, 19, 24, 103
  Relationship Care, 197, 198
  Relationship Check worksheet, 207–208
  Re-Track worksheet, 237–238
  Right Words—SEALS handout, 192
  Safety Plan, 127
  Skills Chain, 85
  Skills Plan, 85, 219
  Solo and Partnership New-Me Activities handout, 145
  Steps of Responsibility worksheet, 213–214
  Summary Sheet, 103
  Switch Tracks to On-Track Action handout, 109
  Take a Step toward My Goal in Wise Mind handout, 106
  Turn the Page handout, 119
  Using My Skills worksheets, 220–224
On-Track Action Plans. *See also* On-Track Action
  Accept the Situation and Turn the Page worksheet, 120–121
  Balancing in My Life worksheet, 115
  Balancing My Life worksheet, 116–117
  Changing Off-Track Relationships handout, 206
  Examples of On-Track Actions worksheet, 122–123
  Five Types of On-Track Actions handout, 105
  My On-Track Action Plan worksheet, 113–114
  On-Track Action Plans handout, 112
  overview, 103
  Relationship Care, 198
On-Track Action Plans handout, 112
On-Track Action: Switching Tracks worksheet, 110–111
On-Track Actions and My Goals worksheet, 107–108
On-Track Relationships, 197, 199. *See also* Relationship Care
On-Track Thinking. *See also* All-the-Time Skills; Check It; Cheerleading; Learning Skills activities; Thoughts; Turn It
  Accept the Situation and Turn the Page worksheet, 120–121
  Categories of Skills handout, 36
  Check It worksheet, 89
  Cheerleading: Blast It worksheet, 94–95
  Clear Picture and, 51
  Expressing Myself, 173
  Expressing Myself Self-Check worksheet, 180
  How Our Skills Help Us handout, 24
  Nine Core Skills handout, 23
  On-Track Action, 103
  On-Track Action: Switching Tracks worksheet, 110–111
  On-Track Thinking: Create a Skills Plan worksheet, 92–93
  On-Track Thinking Through a Situation worksheet, 87–88
  On-Track Thinking to Meet My Goals handout, 86
  overview, 17, 19, 24, 85
  Pros and Cons of Using Skills worksheet, 98–99
  Relationship Care, 197, 198

On-Track Thinking (cont.)
  Relationship Check worksheet, 207–208
  Right Person handout, 189
  Right Tone handout, 191
  Safety Plan, 127
  Skills Chain, 85
  Skills Plan, 85, 219
  Solo and Partnership New-Me Activities handout, 145
  Summary Sheet, 85
  Switch Tracks to On-Track Action handout, 109
  Take a Step toward My Goal in Wise Mind handout, 106
  Turn It worksheet, 90–91
  Turn the Page handout, 119
  Using Skills in My Life worksheet, 96–97
On-Track Thinking: Create a Skills Plan worksheet, 92–93
On-Track Thinking Through a Situation worksheet, 87–88
On-Track Thinking to Meet My Goals handout, 86
Opposite Action, 103, 109, 110–111, 173. *See also* On-Track Action
Outside Risks, 127, 128, 129–130, 136. *See also* Risks
Overrating risk, 127. *See also* Risks

Partnership New-Me Activities. *See also* New-Me Activities
  My Distraction New-Me Activities worksheet, 152
  My Feel Good New-Me Activities worksheet, 150
  My Focus New-Me Activities worksheet, 147
  My Fun New-Me Activities worksheet, 154
  overview, 143
  Solo and Partnership New-Me Activities handout, 145
Pictures in communication, 173, 174. *See also* Communication
Plans A, B, and C, 159, 162, 167–168, 169–170. *See also* Problem Solving
Pre-Learning activities
  Exploring My Goals worksheet, 13–14
  Exploring Targets to Reach My Goal worksheet, 15–16
  Getting to Know Me worksheet, 5–6
  Getting to Know My Feelings worksheet, 7–8
  My Goals worksheet, 11–12
  My New-Me and My Old Me worksheet, 9–10
  overview, 2, 3
Problem Solving. *See also* Calm-Only Skills; Check All Options; Clear Picture of the Problem; Learning Skills activities; Plans A, B, and C
  Categories of Skills handout, 36
  Check All Options worksheet, 165–166
  Clear Picture of the Problem worksheet, 163–164
  Examples of On-Track Actions worksheet, 122–123
  Finding Middle Ground handout, 209
  How Our Skills Help Us handout, 24
  Make Plans A, B, and C worksheet, 167–168
  Nine Core Skills handout, 23
  123 Wise Mind worksheet, 124
  overview, 19, 24, 159, 162
  Problem Solving handout, 162
  Problem Solving Plan worksheet, 169–170
  Quick Fix worksheet, 160–161
  Skills Chain, 85
  Skills Plan, 85, 219
  Summary Sheet, 159
  Take a Step toward My Goal in Wise Mind handout, 106
  Using My Skills worksheets, 220–224
  Why Do I Express Myself? handout, 177
Problem Solving Plan worksheet, 169–170
Progress monitoring, 2, 233–234
Pros and cons, 98–99, 165–166, 169–170, 173
Pros and Cons of Using Skills worksheet, 98–99

Quick Fix, 159, 160–161
Quick Fix worksheet, 160–161

Reaching Goals activities. *See also* Goals
  Back-Track worksheet, 235–236
  My Diary Card worksheet, 231–232
  My Progress worksheet, 233–234
  My Skills Plan worksheet, 229–230
  overview, 2, 227
  Re-Track worksheet, 237–238
Recipe for Skills. *See also* System Tools
  Build Your Recipe for Skills worksheet, 44
  How I Use the Skills System handout, 31
  overview, 19, 31
  Recipe for Skills: Choose How Many Skills to Use worksheet, 42–43
  Recipe for Skills handout, 41
  Review Questions, 47
  Skills Plan, 85
  Week 2 Practice Activity worksheet, 45–46
Recipe for Skills: Choose How Many Skills to Use worksheet, 42–43
Recipe for Skills handout, 41
Relationship Care. *See also* Build On-Track Relationships; Calm-Only Skills; Learning Skills activities; Self-Acceptance; Self-Awareness; Self-Trust; Self-Value
  Balancing On-Track Relationships handout, 203
  Balancing On-Track Relationships: One- and Two-Way Streets handout, 204
  Balancing On-Track Relationships worksheet, 205
  Building, Balancing, and Changing Relationships handout, 199
  Building On-Track Relationships: Different Types of Relationships handout, 202
  Building On-Track Relationships handout, 200
  Building On-Track Relationships worksheet, 201
  Categories of Skills handout, 36
  Changing Off-Track Relationships handouts, 206, 212
  Examples of On-Track Actions worksheet, 122–123
  Expressing Myself, 173
  Finding Middle Ground handout, 209
  Finding Middle Ground Plan worksheet, 210–211
  How Our Skills Help Us handout, 24
  New-Me Activities, 143
  Nine Core Skills handout, 23
  123 Wise Mind worksheet, 124
  overview, 19, 24, 197–198
  Relationship Check worksheet, 207–208
  Skills Chain, 85
  Skills Plan, 85, 219
  Solo and Partnership New-Me Activities handout, 145
  Steps of Responsibility worksheet, 213–214
  Summary Sheet, 197–198
  Take a Step toward My Goal in Wise Mind handout, 106
  Using My Skills worksheets, 220–224
  Why Do I Express Myself? handout, 177
Relationship Check worksheet, 207–208
Re-Track, 237–238
Re-Track worksheet, 237–238
Right Mind, 185, 186, 187, 188. *See also* Getting It Right
Right Mind handout, 187
Right Mind Self-Check worksheet, 188
Right Person, 185, 186, 189. *See also* Getting It Right
Right Person handout, 189
Right Time and Place, 185, 186, 190. *See also* Getting It Right
Right Time and Place handout, 190
Right Tone, 185, 186, 191. *See also* Getting It Right
Right Tone handout, 191
Right Words: SEALS, 173, 185, 186, 192. *See also* Getting It Right
Right Words—SEALS handout, 192
Risks
  Building a Safety Plan worksheet, 136
  Detailed Safety Plan worksheet, 139–140
  Examples of High, Medium, and Low Risks worksheet, 132–133
  Examples of Inside and Outside Risks worksheet, 129–130

Getting a Clear Picture of the Risk: Three Levels of Risk handout, 131
Inside and Outside Risks handout, 128
Safety Plan, 127
Three Ways to Handle Risk handout, 135
Written Safety Plan worksheet, 137–138
Safety Pickle, 127, 135, 139–140. *See also* Safety Plan
Safety Plan. *See also* All-the-Time Skills; Focus on a New-Me Activity; Learning Skills activities; Leave the Area; Move Away; Safety Pickle
Building a Safety Plan worksheet, 136
Categories of Skills handout, 36
Changing Off-Track Relationships handout, 206
Detailed Safety Plan worksheet, 139–140
Examples of High, Medium, and Low Risks worksheet, 132–133
Examples of Inside and Outside Risks worksheet, 129–130
Examples of On-Track Actions worksheet, 122–123
Finding Middle Ground handout, 209
Getting a Clear Picture of the Risk: Three Levels of Risk handout, 131
How Our Skills Help Us handout, 24
Inside and Outside Risks handout, 128
Nine Core Skills handout, 23
123 Wise Mind worksheet, 124
On-Track Action, 103
overview, 19, 24, 127
Problem Solving, 159
Relationship Care, 198
Skills Chain, 85
Skills Plan, 85, 219
Summary Sheet, 127
Take a Step toward My Goal in Wise Mind handout, 106
Three Types of Safety Plans handout, 134
Three Ways to Handle Risk handout, 135
Using My Skills worksheets, 220–224
When Do I Use Expressing Myself? handout, 179
Written Safety Plan worksheet, 137–138
SEALS. *See* Right Words: SEALS
Select the Category of Skills by Feeling Level (worked example 2 and worksheet 3), 38–39
Select the Category of Skills by Feeling Level worksheet, 38–39
Self-Acceptance, 197, 200. *See also* Relationship Care
Self-assessment
Exploring My Goals worksheet, 13–14
Exploring Targets to Reach My Goal worksheet, 15–16
Getting to Know Me worksheet, 5–6

Getting to Know My Feelings worksheet, 7–8
My Goals worksheet, 11–12
My New-Me and My Old Me worksheet, 9–10
Pre-Learning activities, 2, 3
Self-Awareness, 197, 200. *See also* Relationship Care
Self-care
Balancing in My Life worksheet, 115
Balancing My Life worksheet, 116–117
My On-Track Action Plan worksheet, 113–114
New-Me Activities, 143
On-Track Action Plans handout, 112
Solo New-Me Activities and Self-Care worksheet, 155–156
Self-talk. *See* Notice My Thoughts
Self-Trust, 197, 200. *See also* Relationship Care
Self-Value, 197, 200. *See also* Relationship Care
Sensations, 59–60, 61–62, 143. *See also* Body Check
Situations. *See also* Accept the Situation
Accept the Situation and Turn the Page worksheet, 120–121
Accepting the Situation handout, 118
Examples of High, Medium, and Low Risks worksheet, 132–133
Examples of On-Track Actions worksheet, 122–123
Getting a Clear Picture of the Risk: Three Levels of Risk handout, 131
Noticing My Reactions worksheet, 80–81
On-Track Thinking Through a Situation worksheet, 87–88
Pros and Cons of Using Skills worksheet, 98–99
risk and, 127
Situations that Lead to Noticing Thoughts worksheet, 68–69
Situations that Lead to Noticing Urges worksheet, 78–79
Thoughts and Feelings Lead to Urges worksheet, 72–73
Three Ways to Handle Risk handout, 135
Using Skills in My Life worksheet, 96–97
Situations that Lead to Noticing Thoughts worksheet, 68–69
Situations that Lead to Noticing Urges worksheet, 78–79
Skills Certificate, 225
Skills Chain
Getting It Right, 185
How Do I Use Expressing Myself? handout, 178
How I Use the Skills System handout, 31
123 Wise Mind worksheet, 124
overview, 85
Recipe for Skills handout, 41
Relationship Care, 198

Skills List. *See also* Learning Skills activities
How Our Skills Help Us handout, 24
Match the Skill Number and Initial to the Picture worksheet, 26
Name the Skill by Number worksheet, 27
Name the Skill by Picture worksheet, 25
Name the Skills and Categories of Skills worksheet, 37
Nine Core Skills handout, 23
overview, 19
Review Questions, 47
Skills Plan
How I Use the Skills System handout, 31
Learning Skills activities, 19
My Skills Plan worksheet, 229–230
On-Track Action, 103
On-Track Thinking and, 85
On-Track Thinking: Create a Skills Plan worksheet, 92–93
On-Track Thinking Through a Situation worksheet, 87–88
On-Track Thinking to Meet My Goals handout, 86
overview, 2
Pre-Learning activities, 3
Reaching Goals activities, 227
Relationship Check worksheet, 207–208
Re-Track worksheet, 237–238
Using My Skills worksheets, 220–224
Using Skills in My Life (skills quiz and answer sheet), 217–218
Skills Plan Map, 219
Skills System, 1–2, 31
Solo and Partnership New-Me Activities handout, 145
Solo New-Me Activities. *See also* New-Me Activities
Distraction New-Me Activities handout, 151
Feel Good New-Me Activities handout, 149
Focus New-Me Activities handout, 146
My Distraction New-Me Activities worksheet, 152
My Feel Good New-Me Activities worksheet, 150
My Focus New-Me Activities worksheet, 147
My Fun New-Me Activities worksheet, 154
overview, 143
Solo and Partnership New-Me Activities handout, 145
Solo New-Me Activities and Self-Care worksheet, 155–156
Solo New-Me Activities and Self-Care worksheet, 155–156
Steps of Responsibility, 173, 198, 199, 212, 213–214. *See also* Relationship Care

Steps of Responsibility worksheet, 213–214
Surroundings, checking. *See* Check My Surroundings
Switch Tracks. *See also* On-Track Action
  Accept the Situation and Turn the Page worksheet, 120–121
  Examples of On-Track Actions worksheet, 122–123
  Five Types of On-Track Actions handout, 105
  New-Me Activities, 143
  On-Track Action: Switching Tracks worksheet, 110–111
  overview, 103
  Relationship Care, 198
  Solo and Partnership New-Me Activities handout, 145
  Switch Tracks to On-Track Action handout, 109
  When Do I Use Expressing Myself? handout, 179
Switch Tracks to On-Track Action handout, 109
System Tools. *See also* Categories of Skills; Feelings Rating Scale; Learning Skills activities; Recipe for Skills
  Build Your Recipe for Skills worksheet, 44
  Categories of Skills handout, 36
  Feelings Rating Scale with Descriptions handout, 33
  Feelings Rating Scale with Pictures handout, 32
  Feelings Rating Scale worksheet, 34–35
  Feelings Ratings and Categories of Skills worksheet, 40
  How I Use the Skills System handout, 31
  Name the Skills and Categories of Skills worksheet, 37
  overview, 19
  Recipe for Skills: Choose How Many Skills to Use worksheet, 42–43
  Recipe for Skills handout, 41
  Review Questions, 47
  Select the Category of Skills by Feeling Level worksheet, 38–39
  Skills Plan Map, 219
  Week 2 Practice Activity worksheet, 45–46

Take a Step toward My Goal, 103, 105, 107–108, 120–121, 122–123. *See also* Goals; On-Track Action

Take a Step toward My Goal in Wise Mind handout, 106
Talking communication, 173, 174. *See also* Communication
Talking Safety Plan, 127, 134, 136, 139–140. *See also* Safety Plan
Thinking Safety Plan, 127, 134, 136, 139–140. *See also* Safety Plan
Thoughts. *See also* Notice My Thoughts; On-Track Thinking
  Accept the Situation and Turn the Page worksheet, 120–121
  Back-Track worksheet, 235–236
  Cheerleading: Blast It worksheet, 94–95
  Examples of Inside and Outside Risks worksheet, 129–130
  Expressing Myself, 173
  Noticing My Reactions worksheet, 80–81
  Noticing My Thoughts handout, 67
  Noticing Thoughts at Different Feelings Levels worksheet, 70–71
  On-Track Thinking: Create a Skills Plan worksheet, 92–93
  overview, 51
  Situations that Lead to Noticing Thoughts worksheet, 68–69
  Thoughts and Feelings Lead to Urges worksheet, 72–73
  Turn the Page handout, 119
Thoughts and Feelings Lead to Urges worksheet, 72–73
Three Types of Safety Plans handout, 134
Three Ways to Handle Risk handout, 135
Turn It, 85, 90–91, 103, 237–238. *See also* On-Track Thinking
Turn It worksheet, 90–91
Turn the Page, 103, 105, 119, 120–121, 143. *See also* On-Track Action
Turn the Page handout, 119
Two-Way-Street Relationship, 173, 197–198, 199, 204, 205. *See also* Relationship Care
Types of New-Me Activities handout, 144

Underrating risk, 127. *See also* Risks
Urges. *See also* Notice My Urges
  Accept the Situation and Turn the Page worksheet, 120–121
  Action Urges by Feelings Level worksheet, 76–77
  Check It worksheet, 89
  Cheerleading: Blast It worksheet, 94–95
  Detailed Safety Plan worksheet, 139–140
  Examples of Inside and Outside Risks worksheet, 129–130
  Feelings and Their Action Urges worksheet, 74–75
  Noticing My Reactions worksheet, 80–81
  On-Track Thinking: Create a Skills Plan worksheet, 92–93
  On-Track Thinking to Meet My Goals handout, 86
  Situations that Lead to Noticing Urges worksheet, 78–79
  Switch Tracks to On-Track Action handout, 109
  Thoughts and Feelings Lead to Urges worksheet, 72–73
  Turn It worksheet, 90–91
Using My Skills worksheets, 220–224
Using Skills in My Life
  Skills Certificate, 225
  Skills Plan Map, 219
  Using My Skills worksheets, 220–224
  Using Skills in My Life (skills quiz and answer sheet), 217–218
  Using Skills in My Life worksheet, 96–97
Using Skills in My Life worksheet, 96–97

Week 2 Practice Activity worksheet, 45–46
What Is Expressing Myself handout, 174
When Do I Use Expressing Myself? handout, 179
Why Do I Express Myself? handout, 177
Wise Mind
  On- and Off-Tracks handout, 104
  123 Wise Mind worksheet, 124
  On-Track Action, 103
  Problem Solving handout, 162
  Skills Plan, 85
  Take a Step toward My Goal in Wise Mind handout, 106
Worked examples, 1, 2, 3. *See also* individual worksheets
Worksheets, 1, 2, 3. *See also* individual worksheets
Written communication, 173, 174, 178. *See also* Expressing Myself
Written Safety Plan, 127, 134, 136, 137–138, 139–140. *See also* Safety Plan
Written Safety Plan worksheet, 137–138